S0-BYS-762

THE PSYCHOLOGY OF
INSANITY

By BERNARD HART

PSYCHOPATHOLOGY
  *Its Development and its Place in
  Medicine*

THE PSYCHOLOGY OF INSANITY

BY

BERNARD HART

C.B.E., M.D. (LOND.), F.R.C.P. (LOND.)

Fellow of University College, London
Consulting Physician in Psychological Medicine
University College Hospital and
National Hospital, Queen Square, London

FIFTH EDITION

CAMBRIDGE UNIVERSITY PRESS

132.1
H 325 p
c. 2

Published by the Syndics of the Cambridge University Press
Bentley House, 200 Euston Road, London NW1 2DB
American Branch: 32 East 57th Street, New York, N.Y.10022

ISBN: 0 521 05219 X

First published 1912
Second edition 1914
Third edition 1916
Reprinted 1918, 1919 (twice), 1920, 1921, 1922, 1923, 1925,
1928, 1929
Fourth edition 1930
Reprinted 1936, 1941, 1943, 1946, 1949, 1952
Fifth edition 1957
Reprinted 1958, 1974

First printed in Great Britain
by Spottiswoode, Ballantyne & Co. Ltd, Colchester
Reprinted in Great Britain
at the University Printing House, Cambridge
(Brooke Crutchley, University Printer)

BRADFORD COLLEGE

FEB 1 1977

— LIBRARY —

PREFACE TO FIRST EDITION

THIS book lays no claim to be a comprehensive treatise upon the psychology of insanity. The number of independent schools of thought existing at the present day, and the fundamental divergence in their methods of investigation, make it obviously impossible to compress such a treatise into the limits of a small volume. All that has been attempted here is the presentation of certain recent developments in abnormal psychology which have already yielded results of fundamental importance, and which seem to offer an exceptionally promising field for further investigation.

An endeavour has been made to develop the subject-matter of the book in a systematic manner, so that the general principles which it is sought to establish may appear in as clear a light as possible. The adoption of the systematic method in a work of this size, however, renders a somewhat dogmatic mode of presentation inevitable. It is necessary, therefore, to warn the reader that many of the theories to which he will be introduced have not as yet been firmly established, and that they are to be regarded rather as suggestive hypotheses which will ultimately require considerable alteration and improvement.

It must be clearly understood, moreover, that no attempt has been made to cover the whole field of insanity. On the contrary, certain sections of that field have been more or less arbitrarily selected, mainly on the ground that they yield fruitful results to psychological methods of investigation. I confidently anticipate that in the future these methods will have a far wider application, but in the present state of our knowledge it must be frankly admitted that there are whole tracts of insanity in which they have only a very limited utility. This confession is all the more necessary on account of the tendency to unduly extensive generalisation evident in the work of many recent investigators. In view of the enormous complexity of mental processes, and the youthfulness of psychology, it is best to realise that progress must inevitably be slow, and that we must be content to feel our way to the scientific laws of the future.

A very large number of the general principles enunciated in this book are due to the genius of Prof. Freud of Vienna, probably the most original and fertile thinker who has yet entered the field of abnormal psychology. Although, however, I cannot easily express the extent to which I am indebted to him, I am by no means prepared to embrace the whole of the vast body of doctrines which Freud and his followers have now laid down. Much of this is in my opinion unproven, and erected upon an unsubstantial foundation. On the other hand, many of Freud's fundamental principles are becoming more and more widely accepted, and the evidence in their favour is rapidly increasing. In the present volume I have endeavoured to introduce only those principles which have already acquired a satisfactory claim to recognition.

Among many other authorities to whose writings I have had recourse, Dr Jung of Zürich, Prof. Janet of Paris, Prof. Karl Pearson, and the late Prof. Krafft-Ebing must be specially mentioned. Lastly, I am very greatly indebted to Mr W. Trotter's two papers on 'Herd Instinct', published in the *Sociological Review* for 1908 and 1909.

I have to thank Dr Edward Mapother for much valuable assistance in the preparation of the manuscript and the revising of the proofs.

BERNARD HART

September 1912

PREFACE TO FIFTH EDITION

THIS book was first published in 1912 and, although it has since been many times reprinted, no material alteration has been made in the original text. Nor, in the present edition, will any such material alteration be found. Some minor modifications have been incorporated, but these are in the main purely verbal in character. The book therefore remains, and must be judged as, a product of 1912.

In these days of rapid advance in every field of scientific endeavour such a policy requires some justification, and this is no less necessary in the field of psychology, where the growth of the present century has been almost revolutionary in its character and extent. The decision to leave the book in its original form has been based on three grounds. In the first place it is concerned with elementary and general principles which have been relatively unaffected by the advances of subsequent years, because those advances have involved the addition of further stories to the building rather than a remaking of the foundations. In the second place, the development of the subject has been so luxuriant, and the divergencies of thought characterising the different schools have become so marked and so complex, that an attempt to bring the text satisfactorily up-to-date after the lapse of more than forty years would be a formidable task, and one which would practically involve, not a new edition, but a new book. Moreover, such an attempt would completely traverse the very modest aim which it was originally sought to achieve. In the third place, perhaps the most cogent justification for the decision to leave the original text essentially unaltered, is that the constant reprintings, both in this country and America, show that the book has preserved an appeal throughout all these years, in spite of the date which it bears.

It is advisable, however, to amplify the grounds which have been stated. The essential aim of the book when it appeared in 1912 was to illustrate how the 'psychological conception' which had gradually developed round about the turn of the century through the work of Janet to the principles of Freud and Jung, served to illuminate the phenomena both of the normal mind and of mental disorder. That illumination, very apparent and striking to the student who had hitherto been nourished on the somewhat arid psychology of former days, was based on concepts which were fairly simple in their structure, and which have now indeed become largely commonplaces. Moreover, the dynamic principles, which we owe to the genius of Freud, were at that time fairly uniformly held by the analytical school of thought. In that very year of 1912, however, serious rifts developed in that school. Jung and Adler, hitherto enthusiastic exponents of Freud's views, diverged radically both from those views and from each other, and ultimately founded quite independent schools of thought. Nevertheless these divergencies were essentially dependent upon the seeking of deeper concepts than those relatively simple and superficial ones to which this book is mainly confined, and the latter therefore have not been very materially affected.

Although no fundamental change has been made in the original text, there have been some purely verbal alterations in subsequent editions. These are mainly the substitution of 'mental hospital' for 'asylum', of 'insane patient' for 'lunatic', and in many places of 'mental disorder' for 'insanity'. These call for some explanation. In the first place, what I have termed rather unhappily in chapter 1 the 'political conception', and which would perhaps be better termed the 'sociological conception', already far advanced in 1912, has since advanced considerably further. It is now universally accepted that the insane are patients suffering from disease just as much as other patients, and that the prejudices formerly directed against them have no shred of justification. To emphasise this change in attitude the old word 'asylum', whose original meaning was entirely innocent and benevolent but which had acquired sinister associations in the eighteenth and nineteenth centuries, was abandoned in the developments of the present century and replaced by the term 'mental hospital' in which the new attitude to insanity was made clear. The change is further manifested by the fact that in the mental hospital of today a very large number of patients, sometimes the majority, enter the hospital voluntarily and without any legal duress.

Next, one of the aims of the book was to develop the thesis that the insane patient was a fellow-man, that his mental processes were not completely chaotic and inexplicable but only variations or exaggerations of processes to be found in the normal mind. In pursuance of this aim the word 'lunatic', originally the offspring of an absurd superstition and already largely obsolescent in 1912, was deliberately employed in the edition of 1912 to underline the old attitude to insanity which the book sought to pillory. Nowadays, however, there is no need to attack what has become an open door; the term 'lunatic' would be completely out of place, and has therefore been discontinued.

Finally, the substitution in many places of the term 'mental disorder' for 'insanity' has arisen in this way. As has just been explained, an original aim of this book was to show that the mental processes of the insane could be paralleled by examples drawn from the normal mind and from minor mental disorders or, as it may be put, to demonstrate the 'sanity of insanity'. Hence, although it was implied that the processes involved ranged in a continuous series from those occurring in the normal mind through the minor mental disorders to pronounced insanity, the latter term tended unduly to dominate the picture. In later editions, and in response to criticisms that the concepts of the book were as interesting when applied to the normal mind or to the minor disorders, the term 'insanity' was in many places replaced by the general term 'mental disorder' in order to make clear that no sharp lines could be placed between the normal and the minor mental disorders on the one hand, nor on the other hand between the latter and definite insanity, but that we were dealing with a continuous series, with the normal at one end and those gross derangements coming under the head of insanity at the other. This procedure has been adhered to in the present edition.

In the fourth edition an Introduction was incorporated which aimed at describing the historical development of psychopathology from its beginnings to the stage it had reached at the time the book was originally published in 1912, in order that the reader might appreciate the foundations upon which the book was built. The greater part of this Introduction has been included in the present edition, with some modifications and the addition of a few remarks upon the development which has occurred in the subject since the first edition appeared.

BERNARD HART

June 1956

CONTENTS

Prefaces . . . . *page* v

Introduction to Fifth Edition 1

Chapter I   THE HISTORY OF MENTAL DISORDER . . 15

II   THE PSYCHOLOGICAL CONCEPTION OF MENTAL
DISORDER 21

III   THE PHENOMENA OF MENTAL DISORDER . 28

IV   DISSOCIATION 39

V   COMPLEXES 52

VI   CONFLICT 65

VII   REPRESSION 72

VIII   MANIFESTATIONS OF REPRESSED COMPLEXES . 78

IX   PROJECTION 90

X   THE IRRATIONALITY OF THE INSANE . . 96

XI   PHANTASY 106

XII   THE SIGNIFICANCE OF CONFLICT . . 119

Index 125

INTRODUCTION TO FIFTH EDITION

This introduction seeks to put before the reader a general sketch of the history of psychopathology from its beginnings to the position which it held in 1912, in order that he may be able to appreciate the place in the subject of the principles described in this book. It therefore attempts to cover a wider field than is proper to an introduction, and for this reason the uninstructed layman will probably find it more intelligible and useful if it is read after rather than before the book.

DEVELOPMENT OF PSYCHOPATHOLOGY PRIOR TO JANET

Psychopathology, the science which attempts to explain the problems of mental disorder by psychological principles and laws, is of comparatively recent growth, and can hardly be said to have existed before the last quarter of the nineteenth century. The remarkable phenomena produced by Mesmer and the other 'magnetisers' had aroused a widespread interest a hundred years earlier, and later investigators had demonstrated that these phenomena were due, not to the magnets, but to the suggestions communicated by the operator. These 'suggestions' were clearly causes of a psychological order, and it was therefore known that psychological causes were capable of bringing about definite changes in mind and body. Until the time of Charcot (1825–93), however, this conception had not been applied to the problem of disease, and we owe to that investigator the first formulation of the view that certain disorders were due simply to the action of 'ideas'. This statement may be said to have been the foundation stone of modern psychopathology, and it led to a series of investigations which rapidly extended our knowledge and understanding of the so-called 'functional nervous disorders', including hysteria, neurasthenia, and other allied conditions. It was soon appreciated that in this group psychological factors of various kinds played a dominant part in the causation, and an attempt began to be made to formulate that part in exact terms. Amongst the psychological factors concerned an important place had clearly to be assigned to 'suggestion', that is to say, the implantation in the patient's mind of certain ideas and beliefs, and their resultant effect in the production of various symptoms and disturbances. Suggestion, however, was a process so vague and general that it could not furnish a really satisfactory explanation of complex disorders, and investigators sought to discover further psychological laws which would render the incidence and nature of these disorders more intelligible, and which would moreover also explain how suggestion produced its results.

WORK OF JANET

The first noteworthy advance in this direction was made by Janet with his conception of 'dissociation'. This conception, which is described in chapter IV of the book, was developed at the end of last century as the result of a brilliant series of researches, and it forms a milestone of fundamental importance in the progress of psychopathology. Janet showed that consciousness does not necessarily consist in a single and homogeneous stream, but that it is sometimes split into a number of more or less independent currents, and that the dissociation thereby produced explains a large number of phenomena, not only in hysteria and other disorders, but in the processes of our everyday mental life. This conception has proved to be extraordinarily fertile as a weapon of understanding, but it is only capable of taking us a certain distance along the road. The further question naturally arises as to why dissociations take place, and the conception of dissociation in itself furnishes no answer to this question. Such an answer will only be forthcoming if we can obtain a knowledge of the dynamics of the mind, that is to say, a knowledge of the forces which produce the various phenomena of mental process and the laws of their action.

The first consistent attempt to advance to a dynamic point of view was made by Freud, who is unquestionably the dominating figure in modern psychopathology, though the precise value and reliability of the vast structure which he has now erected is still a matter of doubt and dispute. The principles described in the later chapters of this book are in the main directly due to him, and for the rest have been developed from the new points of view which his genius originated. Nevertheless the angle of approach to the subject and the method of treatment in the book diverged even at the time of its publication in many important respects from the path followed by Freud. Freud's later work has tended to accentuate these divergences, while it has added much new knowledge and even more new theory to the original structure. His doctrines now occupy so prominent a place in modern psychology, moreover, that they demand consideration, not merely as a contribution to the building of our subject, but as a more or less complete system of thought, laying down its own postulates and laws, and relatively independent of other modes of approach. For these reasons, therefore, it is necessary that the reader of this book should appreciate the mode and extent in which its viewpoint differed from Freud's position as it stood in 1912, and the development which his work has undergone in the years which have since elapsed. An attempt to achieve this purpose will be made by giving here a brief summary of Freud's views in their historical perspective; but such a sketch must necessarily be very inadequate, and it is hoped that it will be amplified by reference to the special literature of the subject.

THE DEVELOPMENT OF FREUD'S CONCEPTIONS

In 1880 Josef Breuer of Vienna investigated a case of hysteria in which he found that the symptoms were due to certain memories of which the patient was herself unconscious, and that a cure was effected when these memories were brought once more into consciousness. Freud collaborated with Breuer in further work along the lines which this discovery suggested, and from that moment he developed gradually but continuously the great structure of theory and practice which is now associated with his name.

It will be noted that almost from the beginning certain fundamental principles were already apparent. These principles were, firstly, that the mind contained more than consciousness, and that memories could exist and continually produce effects, although those memories were divorced from and inaccessible to consciousness. The mind therefore consisted not only of conscious but also of unconscious processes. Secondly, the memories shut out from consciousness must be subjected to some force which actively prevented their appearance in consciousness, for they were not capable of being recalled by any ordinary means. This active force was termed 'resistance', and it was a plausible inference that the force which did not permit of the excluded memories entering consciousness had originally been responsible for that very exclusion.

The next step was the determination of the way in which this exclusion, or 'repression' as it was technically termed, arose and why it was being maintained. Investigation led Freud to conclude that repression occurred because of the simultaneous existence in the mind of two incompatible strivings and the attempt of the mind to get rid of this intolerable strain by excluding one of the opponents from consciousness. This opponent then passed into the unconscious regions of the mind, where it was still capable of activity but could not directly appear upon the conscious stage. The situation could therefore now be depicted in this way. The hysterical symptoms, for example paralyses or anaesthesias, were produced by mental factors which were unconscious but active; they were unconscious because they had been incompatible with other forces in the mind and had been repressed from consciousness as a method of avoiding the conflict which was otherwise inevitable. The symptoms thus served to express,

4

albeit in an indirect and distorted manner, a striving which although existing in the mind was not allowed to appear in consciousness. The distortion was due to the repressing forces, and the symptoms could therefore be said to constitute the end-product produced by the interaction of the repressed and repressing forces.

The various ways in which this interaction occurred were worked out in detail, and a number of 'mechanisms' were formulated which described the mode in which the forces concerned caused the appearance of a 'symptom'. Several of these mechanisms are dealt with in the pages of this book (chapters VIII and IX).

It was found, moreover, not only that the processes which were being discovered were to be discerned in hysteria, but also that they were responsible for the symptoms observed in other types of nervous and mental disorder, and were capable of explaining many of the psychological phenomena of everyday life. The investigation of dreams proved to be particularly fruitful in this respect, and led to the discovery that their structure and mode of development were essentially analogous to those observed in the production of neurotic symptoms. This discovery was of great practical importance, because it was found that a study of the dreams of a patient enabled the investigator to elucidate the nature of the forces acting in the mind, and hence could be used as a method of ascertaining the facts necessary for the patient's treatment.

It has been mentioned that Freud's theories involved the assumption that the mind did not only consist of consciousness, but that it also comprised processes of which the individual himself was completely unaware, although they were capable of activities otherwise comparable with those observed in consciousness. This assumption of the existence of an unconscious mind was elaborated by Freud into a new conception of mental topography. He held that three regions existed in the mind—the conscious, the foreconscious, and the unconscious. In the conscious region were contained those processes which comprise consciousness in the ordinary sense of the term. In the foreconscious were processes which, though not conscious at the moment, might immediately become so by a simple act of recall. In the unconscious were processes which not only were not conscious at the moment, but could not become so by any ordinary means. Between the unconscious and the other regions was a barrier which allowed no direct passage, but through which the unconscious processes could obtain egress provided that they underwent modification and distortion. It will be seen that the passage from the other regions to the unconscious constituted 'repression', and that the barrier just described constituted the resistance and distorting medium which we have already observed in the mechanism of symptoms.

In working out the various ways in which the forces interacting in the mind produced the phenomena of dreams and the symptoms of nervous disorder Freud naturally investigated the nature and origin of the forces concerned. He found that forces derived from the sex instincts invariably played a part therein, and in order to explain these facts he gradually developed the elaborate sexual theory which has become the kernel of his doctrines.

Freud held that sex as we know it in the adult was the final stage of a long process of evolution, which commenced in earliest infancy. During this evolution it underwent considerable changes, so that the adult manifestations were radically different from the infantile, although the driving force or 'libido' remained essentially the same throughout. In the initial stages the libido was directed on to the individual himself; later it became capable of being directed on to external objects. The first of these external objects was generally one or other parent, predominantly the parent of the opposite sex. Later still the object of the libido was constituted by an individual of the same sex, and only at the final stage did it attain the normal adult character, and become directed on to individuals of the opposite sex. The libido was thus conceived to pass through a succession of phases, autoerotic, parental, homosexual, and heterosexual. This development in the object

6

relationship of the libido was paralleled by an alteration in the parts of the body with which it was particularly associated.

Freud believed that this lengthy development of the libido could miscarry in various ways, and that if such miscarriage occurred perversions or disorders were produced. If the development failed to proceed beyond the homosexual stage one form of sexual perversion was manifested. If the change from one stage to the next was not properly completed, so that the libido remained partially attached or 'fixated' to an earlier object relationship, while partially moving forwards to the normal adult goal, then a state of conflict was produced, with the repression into the unconscious of these partially developed elements of the libido, and the resultant appearance of neurotic disorder.

It has been said that Freud found that forces derived from the sex instincts invariably played a part in the conflicts and interactions responsible for the phenomena of dreams and neurotic disorder or, as we may now express it, that an activity of the libido was necessarily involved. Freud observed, however, that forces of an apparently quite different kind were also concerned. These latter forces belonged to the personality or governing body of the organism, and collectively formed the 'ego'; the ego would not permit the libido to pursue an untrammelled course, because control and inhibition were necessary in the interests of that adaptation to the demands of reality and environment which constituted the ego's chief function. Investigation showed, indeed, that the conflicts underlying the symptoms of nervous disorder were essentially due to the struggle between the libido and the ego or, as Freud himself later expressed it, a nervous disorder develops 'when the Ego loses its capacity to deal in some way or other with the Libido'. If this situation should occur, then conflict would necessarily arise, and the attempt of the organism to solve this conflict would lead to repressions, and the appearance of 'symptoms' in the way which has already been described.

Something must now be said of the method of investigation which Freud employed in building up his theories. This was the method of 'psychoanalysis', and it of course constitutes the keystone of the whole structure. The method was developed as a means of obtaining access to the unconscious mental processes which Freud believed to be responsible for the symptoms observed in his patients. Clearly, as these processes were by hypothesis unconscious, they could not be elicited by simple inquiry or observation, and some special procedure had to be devised. In his earliest researches Freud had used hypnotism for this purpose, as it had long been known that by this means access could be obtained to mental elements of which the individual was completely unaware. Later, however, it was found that the unconscious processes could be elicited by a method more widely applicable than hypnotism, and more fertile in its results. Freud noted that if the patient were asked to talk freely without making any attempt to control or direct the course of his thoughts, then these thoughts were determined in part by unconscious factors, and the skilled investigator could conclude from the character of the thoughts the nature of the causal unconscious processes. Freud termed this method 'psychoanalysis', and gradually developed it into an elaborate weapon for the investigation and treatment of mental disorder. The whole of his work, including all the theories developed in later years, is based upon its employment, and the facts which have been elicited by its means.

Freud's earlier researches were mainly concerned with nervous disorders, but he had noted that processes closely comparable to those found in these disorders were also to be discerned in certain forms of insanity. This path was further explored by Jung, at that time a follower of Freud, although he has since developed an altogether independent school of thought. Jung's investigation of dementia praecox, one of the most common forms of mental disorder, produced results of the first importance, and demonstrated that the psychological laws which Freud had discovered in his study of hysteria played a prominent part in dementia praecox, although of course fundamental differences existed between the two disorders.

The point which we have now reached corresponds roughly to the stage in Freud's development which had been achieved at the time of the publication of this book. It has, of course, only been possible to attempt a brief and inadequate sketch of the essential structure of Freud's theories, which had even at that time already attained a great complexity, but it is hoped that a sufficiently clear picture will have been given to indicate broadly the road along which he had travelled in his investigations. If this aim has been successfully achieved the reader will have no difficulty in understanding the points in which the treatment of the subject in this book differs from that followed by Freud.

In the first place, there is a notable difference in the angle of approach. Freud slowly and tentatively built up his theoretical conceptions in accordance with the facts which were continuously elicited by his investigation of patients, and he made no attempt to produce a systematic exposition of the subject as a whole. In other words, he did not produce textbooks, but a series of monographs. In this book, on the other hand, a systematic exposition has been attempted, and the principles described have therefore been set out, not in their historical perspective, but in accordance with the place which belongs to them in that exposition. Moreover, the subject has been treated in a way which seeks constantly to demonstrate that the conceptions of psychopathology are constructed according to the rules which govern all progress in science, or, in other words, that they conform to the canons of scientific method. For this reason many of Freud's conceptions have been dealt with from a philosophical standpoint which does not correspond to the angle from which he himself had reached them, and which is in some respects not entirely compatible with that angle.

In the second place, the book does not profess to be a description of Freud's theories. It covers only a small part of the field which Freud has tilled, and many of the most important sections of his work are not even mentioned. Moreover, it includes such conceptions as dissociation, which either lie outside his line of development or have only played a small and relatively unimportant part therein.

As a result of these two main lines of divergence certain of Freud's conceptions are treated in this book in a way which does not correspond to the place and importance they possess in the building up of his system. For example, Freud's topographical differentiation of the mind into conscious, preconscious, and unconscious regions has not been adopted. The existence of unconscious processes has been assumed as a conception necessary for the adequate explanation of the phenomena of consciousness, but these processes are regarded from a functional rather than a topographical standpoint, and they have not the precise and peculiar character which Freud ascribes to his 'Unconscious'.

Another example is furnished by the omission from the book of any detailed consideration of the sex instincts. Freud's view that the sex instincts play a fundamental part in the conflicts responsible for various disorders is indeed mentioned, but it is merely put forward as a possible hypothesis concerning the nature of the ultimate factors involved. In Freud's own work, on the other hand, this hypothesis has been present almost from the beginning, and the development and activity of the libido has formed the central structure round which all his theories have been built.

It must be understood, therefore, that this book does not really occupy any definite place in the direct line of Freudian history, but is at once narrower and wider in its aim; narrower in that it only deals with certain selected aspects of Freud's teaching, and wider in that it attempts to bring those aspects into relation with the lines of advance followed by other investigators.

DEVELOPMENT OF PSYCHOPATHOLOGY SINCE 1912

It has been explained in the Preface that any attempt to bring the book up-to-date by amending the text, or by describing, however briefly, the development and growth of the subject during the past forty years, would not only be an impossible task within any reasonable limits but would inevitably destroy the very modest aim which the book sought to achieve. No such attempt will be made here, but this Introduction may well be concluded by some general remarks concerning the subsequent fate of the principles which the book describes.

The dominating feature of the history of the first half of the present century has been the increasing influence exerted by the works of Freud. This influence has extended far beyond the limits of the orthodox psychoanalytical school, and it is not too much to say that his conceptions have profoundly affected the course of nearly all modern psychopathological investigation. This statement does not mean that there has been a general acceptance of the vast structure of theory and practice which Freud has erected. On the contrary, the validity of that structure is still a subject of more or less acrimonious dispute, and Freud's doctrines are embraced in their entirety only by a relatively small school of thought composed of his immediate followers, and constituting what we have termed the orthodox school of psychoanalysis. The new avenues of approach to psychological problems which Freud first opened, however, the weapons which he devised for his investigations, and the supremely important establishment of a dynamic outlook in research, all these have fundamentally modified the whole subsequent history of psychopathology. Moreover, a considerable number of Freud's earlier conceptions—in particular the notion of conflict and the various 'mechanisms' whereby conflict produces the phenomena of neurotic disorder—have attained a wide recognition, and are indeed within a measurable degree of general acceptance.

The orthodox school of psychoanalysis, mainly under the direct leadership of its founder, has developed the method of psychoanalysis into an elaborate and complex weapon of investigation, and has extended its researches into ever-widening fields. In addition to the sphere of nervous disorder, which was the subject of Freud's earlier work, normal psychology, sociology, anthropology, and education have been successively attacked. It may indeed be said that the Freudian doctrines have developed into a more or less complete and self-contained system of thought, seeking to solve the problems of life and mind along its own lines, and with but little contact or co-operation with other methods of approach.

In this development Freud's earlier conceptions have been generally maintained, but they have sustained an extensive elaboration. The growth and mutations of the libido have been traced out in great detail, and the factors formerly grouped roughly together as the 'ego' have been analysed into several components, each possessing definite characters and functions. In the interaction of these components and those of the libido an explanation has been sought of the phenomena of normal and morbid mental life, and the explanation has been pushed into almost every sphere of psychological and biological activity.

It has been pointed out that the influence of Freud's work has extended far beyond the orthodox school of psychoanalysis, and certain of his conceptions have been incorporated in the work of many other psychopathologists who are not prepared to accept Freud's views in their entirety. Two schools of thought call for special mention here, founded respectively by Jung and Adler. These investigators were formerly followers of Freud, but their lines of advance have diverged widely from the path of orthodox psychoanalysis. Both Jung and Adler have availed themselves of the new avenues opened up by Freud and have to some extent adopted certain of his conceptions, but each has proceeded along a separate road, and has produced an almost completely independent body of doctrine and practice.

The divergencies between these two schools, and indeed those between all the various competing schools of psychopathology at the present day, are essentially dependent upon the seeking of deeper concepts than those relatively simple and superficial ones to which this book is mainly confined, and the latter therefore have not been very materially affected.

It may be remarked that the divergencies which seem inevitably to occur when an attempt is made to formulate deeper concepts are a characteristic illustration of a fundamental weakness of the psychological method of approach in comparison with that employed by other sciences, notably physics. In chapter II it is explained that the method of science consists in three steps, firstly the collection and recording of phenomena, secondly the classification of these phenomena into series or sequences, and thirdly the discovery of a short formula which will enable us to describe these sequences in the most comprehensive and convenient manner. This third step not only provides a formula which permits of the facts observed being resumed, but it should also permit of our predicting other sequences of phenomena, particularly those resulting from controlled experiments. It is in the attempt to fulfil the third step completely that the relative weakness of the psychological conception appears. In physics no theoretical construction would be accepted as valid unless it served not only to resume the facts observed, but also enabled us to predict without failure the course of other sequences experimentally controlled. Now psychological theories can be constructed to resume or explain observed facts, but it is rarely possible, except in the case of comparatively simple processes, to carry out that decisive part of the third step, the predicting of the results which will be achieved by experimental investigation of further sequences. Hence the ground is left free for different psychopathologists to devise different theoretical constructions, which do in fact serve to resume and explain the phenomena observed, but which are mutually incompatible. The conclusive test in deciding between them, namely, their capacity to predict with certainty the course of other sequences of phenomena, particularly of phenomena experimentally regulated, is, to a great extent, lacking, at any rate with regard to the phenomena dealt with in this book. Hence divergent schools of thought unfortunately but inevitably arise.

The attack on the problems of mental disorder is nowadays

being conducted on a very wide front. Apart from the approaches which stem wholly or in part from the work of Freud, psychologists are carrying out investigations which employ experimental, mathematical, and statistical methods, and which seek to remain strictly within the canons of scientific research. The problems of human behaviour, both normal and morbid, are being examined by many authorities with the aid of concepts built differently from those of the analytical psychopathologists, and with the help of contributions culled from such ancillary sciences as sociology and anthropology.

Finally there have been great developments within what is described in chapter II as the 'physiological conception', i.e. the view that mental phenomena are manifestations of processes taking place in the brain and other organs, with the resultant corollary that the search for fundamental causes must be directed to those physical processes. These developments have not so far resulted in demonstrating satisfactorily the anatomical, physiological and chemical changes which underlie the phenomena of insanity, though some progress has been made in this direction, but lie in the field of treatment. In recent years direct attack upon the brain by electrical and operative measures has proved remarkably fruitful in dealing with certain disorders. It is not unreasonable to suppose that, when the physiological and other changes responsible for these results have been discovered, they will fall within a physiological rather than a psychological conception.

CHAPTER I

THE HISTORY OF MENTAL DISORDER

RECORDS of abnormal mental phenomena reach back to the very dawn of history, and are to be found in the oldest books in both the Eastern and the Western world. Thus, in the Old Testament we read of Saul's recurring periods of depression, when 'the evil spirit from the Lord' was upon him. We read, again, of the delirium of Nebuchadnezzar, in which he believed himself changed into an animal—he 'did eat grass like an ox, and his body was wet with the dew of heaven, till his hairs grew like the feathers of eagles, and his nails like birds' claws'. To turn to the West, abnormal mental phenomena frequently appear in the pages of Homer. Ajax was tortured by the Furies till he fell upon his own sword, and we are told that Ulysses simulated madness in order to justify his abstention from the Trojan war. The famous oracles are not altogether attributable to fraud, but are probably partly to be explained as hysterical manifestations similar to those found in the 'medium' of the present day.

Side by side with the abnormal phenomenon we invariably find its attempted explanation, because the demand for explanation is a fundamental character of the human mind. Throughout the history of mental disorder, and particularly with regard to the more severe forms of mental disorder comprised under the term 'insanity', this demand constantly makes itself felt, endeavouring to obtain satisfaction by the construction of explanations in harmony with the general thought and knowledge of the period. These attempted explanations we shall know as the various 'conceptions of mental disorder', and the aim of the present chapter will be to trace their historical development until we reach the modern 'psychological conception of mental disorder', with which this book as a whole is mainly concerned.

15

Now the conception of mental disorder to be found in those ancient records mentioned above may be described as the 'demonological'. The phenomena were regarded as the manifestations of some spiritual being, god or demon, who either actually inhabited the body of his victim, or who merely played upon him from without. If the phenomena manifested were in harmony with the religious views of the time it was concluded that the controlling spirit was benign in character, and the individual possessed was revered as an exceptionally holy person. If, on the other hand, the individual's conduct conflicted with the dominating ethical code, he was thought to be the victim of a malignant devil. So long as this view was generally accepted, it was natural that the only curative treatment in force was the employment of religious ceremonials and incantations.

With the coming of Hippocrates, however, somewhere about the year 460 B.C., the conception of insanity in Greece underwent a radical change. Hippocrates, the father of medicine, laid down the principle that the brain was the organ of mind, and that insanity was merely the result of some disturbance in this organ. He 'led his patients out of the temple of Æsculapius and proceeded to treat them along the lines of ordinary medicine'.

This view, the first attempt to attack insanity by the method of science, was not destined at that time to any very fruitful development, and it disappeared altogether in the intellectual stagnation of the Dark Ages. Medieval Europe shows us the subordination of thought, literature, and art to the service of an all-powerful church, the replacement of philosophy by scholasticism, and of science by mysticism.

The prevailing views upon the nature and causation of insanity reverted, as a natural consequence, to the demonological conception of the ancients. The doctrine that abnormal mental symptoms were the product of a supernatural agency, holy or evil, again made its appearance, and attained in the Middle Ages to its extreme development.

In the records of the ascetics and ecstatics who flourished at that period we find manifestations constantly described, visions and trances for example, which are of frequent occurrence in the mentally disordered patient of today. The current beliefs of the Middle Ages, however, regarded such phenomena as the result of an intimate communion with the Deity, and the individuals in whom they occurred were correspondingly revered and esteemed.

A number of other abnormal mental phenomena were grouped together under the conception of 'witchcraft', one of the most characteristic products of medieval thought. The age of witchcraft presents a fascinating chapter of human history, still replete with unsolved problems. It is very probable, however, that many of the rites of witchcraft, the witches' sabbath and other feasts, were relics of the prehistoric religion of Europe, the religion of German mythology. They therefore formed, as it were, a cult persisting alongside the dominating religion of the day. Now cults of this character inevitably attract to their ranks numerous recruits from the army of the mentally unstable, a fact which we can see constantly exemplified in our own time. Hence it is not surprising that we find amongst the witches numbers of people who would now be definitely classed as neurotic or insane. Certain signs which are well known to the modern physician as symptoms of hysteria became, indeed, regarded as indisputable proofs that a particular individual was a witch. One such sign was the famous 'devil's claw', a patch of insensitive skin somewhere upon the body of the alleged witch, a sign frequently met with in the modern hospital under the less lurid name of 'hysterical anaesthesia'. The determination of the existence of the 'devil's claw', together with a number of other fantastic tests, constituted the procedure of the witch-trial. This atrocious institution obtained a firm hold upon the nations of Europe, and persisted even into the eighteenth century. Some idea of its extent may be gained from the fact that within a few years six thousand five hundred people were executed for witchcraft in the principality of Trèves alone.

Those abnormal mental phenomena which could be

ascribed neither to holiness nor to witchcraft were mostly thought to be due to the agency of malignant demons. The unfortunate individuals who exhibited them were subjected to exorcism and other ceremonials and, if this treatment failed to produce a cure, they were cast into dungeons, or ostracised from society.

The reform of this very unsatisfactory state of affairs was due to the development of two distinct lines of thought— science and humanitarianism. The method of science, which was soon to revolutionise human knowledge, was in its early days almost solely devoted to the study of the material world. The objective mode of thought which this study induced, however, could not but have far-reaching effects, and with the decay of scholasticism came the decay of the demonological conception of insanity. Finally, modern Europe attained to that stage which Hippócrates had reached more than a thousand years before. Mental phenomena were thought to be manifestations of processes taking place in the brain, and the principle was laid down that insanity was a disease of the brain, just as pneumonia was a disease of the lungs. At the beginning of the nineteenth century, therefore, we find the modern 'physiological conception' of insanity definitely established.

This stage was preceded by a transition period dominated by what may be termed the 'political conception'. Although the insane were no longer regarded as the peculiar property of the devil, it was thought that they had no claim upon the consideration of society. So long as the madman was prevented from troubling his fellow-men, the community felt that every duty had been discharged. This was the epoch of dungeons and chains.

Men covered with filth cowered in cells of stone, cold, damp, without air or light, and furnished with a straw bed that was rarely renewed, and which soon became infectious—frightful dens where we should scruple to lodge the vilest animals. The insane thrown into these receptacles were at the mercy of their attendants, and these attendants were convicts from prison. The unhappy patients were loaded with chains and bound like galley slaves.

The revolting misery of the asylums of those days has been pictured by the hand of Hogarth; it can hardly be described in words.

The first work of humanitarianism in the field of insanity stands to the credit of England. In the reform of St Luke's in London, towards the end of the eighteenth century, and the foundation of the Retreat in York, we meet with the first serious attempt to better the material circumstances of the insane. Dr Conolly at Hanwell abolished the chains which had been hitherto an essential feature of every asylum, and similar reforms were carried out in France under the leadership of Pinel and Esquirol. Since those days the humanitarian movement has made continuous progress, the right of the insane to be treated as human beings is now universally recognised, and the mental hospital of today has become a model of comfort and orderliness.

This advance in the methods of administration and treatment has been helped at every step by the parallel advance of science. By the end of the eighteenth century the view that abnormal mental phenomena must be attacked along the lines which had everywhere else led to a material advance in knowledge had attained a firm hold, and at that period the foundations were laid of a genuine scientific study of insanity. This study, constituting the branch of science known as psychiatry, has undergone a great development during the past hundred years, and a considerable body of knowledge has now been accumulated.

We have seen that at the beginning of the nineteenth century, the physiological conception had attained almost universal acceptance. Research began to be devoted mainly to the anatomy and physiology of the brain, and our knowledge of these subjects increased at an extraordinarily rapid rate. With the aid of the microscope the anatomical structure of the brain was worked out in its most minute details, and the application of experimental methods to cerebral physiology led to still further advances. Chief amongst the latter was the demonstration of the facts of cerebral topography, the discovery that definite portions of the brain controlled definite bodily functions. It was found, for example, that a portion of the brain, now known as the 'motor area', controlled all the movements of the head and limbs, so that if a part of this area were destroyed, complete paralysis of the corresponding limb immediately followed.

In the enthusiasm created by these discoveries it was confidently anticipated that the nature and causes of mental disorder would speedily be laid bare. These hopes have not been realised, however, and the opinion is rapidly gaining ground that, although the value of the physiological method cannot be disputed, there is ample room for some other mode of approaching the problem. This other mode has now been furnished by the development of the 'psychological conception'.

The psychological conception is based on the view that mental processes can be directly studied without any reference to the accompanying changes which are presumed to take place in the brain, and that mental disorder may therefore be properly attacked from the standpoint of psychology. Early attempts to develop this aspect were largely vitiated by the confusion of psychology with metaphysics, theology, and ethics. We find, for example, Heinroth maintaining that insanity was the result of sin, and could only be cured by the attainment of religious faith. Finally, however, psychology succeeded in freeing itself from its alien companions, and the way was clear for its application to the study of mental disorder. The first great advances in this direction were made by the French psychologists during the latter half of the nineteenth century, culminating in the classical work of Janet. In recent years progress has been rapid, and with the researches of Kraepelin, Freud, and Jung, the psychological conception of mental disorder has become a recognised avenue of explanation and attack.

At the present day, therefore, there are two dominating 'conceptions', the physiological and the psychological, differing widely in their mode of dealing with the subject, but both alike founded upon the employment of the scientific method.

CHAPTER II

THE PSYCHOLOGICAL CONCEPTION OF MENTAL DISORDER

It is necessary that we should clearly understand what is meant by the psychological conception of mental disorder, the relation it bears to the physiological conception, and the nature of its aims and methods. The consideration of these problems involves some preliminary acquaintance with the fundamental propositions upon which modern science is based, and inevitably leads to questions which are, strictly speaking, beyond the limits of our subject. But as no clear thinking in psychology is possible unless precise notions about these elementary matters have been previously acquired, we may perhaps be pardoned for temporarily trespassing upon the domain of philosophy.

It has been pointed out that modern science is attacking the problem of mental disorder along two different routes. The psychological conception treats the phenomena as states of mind, whereas the physiological conception treats them merely as manifestations of changes occurring in the brain. Now in this statement we are confronted with certain terms which, although loosely and erroneously used in ordinary language, have nevertheless a precise and definite signification. These terms are 'science', 'mind', 'brain', 'physiology', and 'psychology'.

Everybody is aware that science is a method of acquiring knowledge, but everybody is not aware that this method is always one and the same, whatever the subject may be to which it is being applied. The scientist who devotes himself to psychology proceeds in exactly the same manner as the scientist who devotes himself to chemistry. The universal method of science consists in certain definite steps, and its nature

B

will be best understood by the consideration of a simple example.[1]

Let us take the process by which we have attained our knowledge of the motion of the planetary system. In the earlier days of astronomy efforts were made to explain this motion by the invention of numerous fantastic hypotheses, but with the advent of Copernicus, Tycho Brahe, and Kepler, these hypotheses were abandoned, and the problem was attacked by the slow but sure method of science. The first step was the laborious collection of the necessary facts. The position of a certain planet in the heavens was carefully observed on a certain day, and the observation repeated at intervals on various subsequent days. These observations were duly classified and in this way a record of the successive positions occupied by the planet during its course was finally obtained. The next step was the discovery of a convenient formula by which these successive positions could be shortly and adequately described. It was discovered by Kepler that if we assume each planet to move around the sun in a certain curve, known to mathematicians as an ellipse, it will be found that our assumption is in precise agreement with the previously collected facts. Thus, knowing the planet's position on 1 January, and knowing its rate of motion, we could calculate how far it would have moved along the ellipse by 14 January. If we then turned to our recorded observation of the planet's position on 14 January, we should find that the calculated position and the position determined by actual observation were in precise agreement. As this test is invariably satisfied, Kepler's formula has been admitted to the rank of a scientific law.

If we analyse the procedure by which this law was ultimately reached, we find that it consists of three successive steps : (1) the collection and recording of facts; (2) the classification of these facts into series or sequences; (3) the discovery of a short formula, or 'scientific law', which will enable us to describe these sequences of facts in the most comprehensive and con-

[1] For the conception of the method of science developed in this chapter the author is mainly indebted to Prof. Karl Pearson's *Grammar of Science*.

venient manner. This is the method of science, and whatever the subject may be, it is the sole method which science ever employs.

Let us now examine another example of the scientific method, the discovery of the various laws constituting the early history of the atomic theory. It is at once clear that the chemist has proceeded by the same three steps which we found in the case of Kepler's planetary law. Firstly the ascertaining of the facts, represented here by the observation of chemical substances, and of the manner in which they decompose or combine together in bulk. Secondly the classification of the facts into series, whereby it is found that in this decomposition and combination the proportion of the constituent substances is always the same. Thirdly the construction of a scientific law designed to explain these facts. This third step was carried out by Dalton; he conceived the hypothesis that chemical substances are composed of minute elements or 'atoms', and that these atoms combine together according to certain simple principles. He found that the formulae thus obtained, constituting in their totality the well-known 'atomic theory', enabled him not only to explain all the facts of chemical combination and decomposition which had already been ascertained by experiment, but also to predict what would happen in any further experiments of a similar kind. Dalton's theory has been subjected to innumerable tests, and it has been found always to agree with the facts of experience. The formulae composing it are therefore, like Kepler's ellipses, now regarded as established scientific laws. The theory is, indeed, so universally recognised and taught, it is so immensely useful, and it explains so much, that the lay reader is in danger of falling into error concerning its true character.

Although Kepler's ellipses and Dalton's atomic theory have both been attained by the use of the scientific method, yet there is an important distinction between them. In the second example a new factor has appeared; we find that Dalton not only constructed a scientific law, but invented the objects between which the law is conceived to hold. He did not know that atoms had any real existence at all. Atoms were merely constructions of the scientific imagination. Precisely similar statements apply to the wave theory of light; the ether and its waves had never been actually observed, they were invented by the scientist in order to explain the facts of light and heat. But their actual non-existence did not in the least vitiate the value which they had for science. They enabled us to resume and predict a vast number of facts, and this is the sole justification which scientific law is ever required to possess.

The distinction which underlies these remarks is expressed in the terms 'phenomenal' and 'conceptual'. 'Phenomena' are facts of experience, things which can be actually observed. 'Concepts' are inventions of the scientist, designed to resume, or in other words, to *explain* the facts of experience. For example, chemical substances and coloured objects are phenomena, atoms and ether waves are concepts.

We are now in a position to complete our description of the method of science. It consists in (1) the observation and recording of the phenomena; (2) the classification of the recorded phenomena into groups or series; (3) the discovery of a formula which will enable us to resume these series in the most comprehensive and convenient manner. The formula may be altogether conceptual in character, that is to say, it may avail itself of imaginary objects whose real existence in nature cannot be demonstrated. The only test which it is required to satisfy is the test of utility, it must explain the facts which we actually find, and it must enable us to predict the occurrence of future facts. If, then, the study of mental disorder is to be made worthy of the name of science, this is the method which must be employed, and the broad lines of the task before us are now clear. A further difficulty, however, remains to be solved. If there is but one method of research, what is the distinction between the physiological conception and the psychological conception?

The physiological conception admits that the phenomena of mental disorder are phenomena of consciousness, but it assumes that the mental processes are accompanied by corre-

24

sponding changes in the brain, and to these brain changes it devotes all its attention. With the phenomena as facts of consciousness it has no immediate concern. The first aim of the physiological conception is to find the actual changes in the brain which occur in mental disorder and the brain changes correlated with each morbid mental process. Its ultimate aim is the discovery of convenient 'laws' which will describe these brain processes in the shortest and most comprehensive manner. These laws will, of course, contain nothing but physiological terms—terms of *consciousness* will find no place therein.

The psychological conception, on the other hand, takes from the outset an altogether different route. It regards the conscious processes occurring in mental disorder as the actual phenomena with which it is called upon to deal. Its ultimate aim is the discovery of convenient 'laws' which will shortly and comprehensively describe these *conscious processes*. In this case the laws will contain nothing but psychological terms—terms of *brain* will find no place therein.

It is of the utmost importance that, in the final 'laws' obtained by either the physiological or the psychological conception, there should be no mixing of the terms. The physiological laws must contain no psychological terms, and the psychological laws must contain no physiological terms. Nothing but hopeless confusion can result from the mixture of 'brain-cells' and 'ideas'. The reader must be asked to accept this statement as a dogma. Any adequate demonstration of its truth would take us far beyond the limits of this book.[1]

The determination of the ultimate relation which the

---

[1] This rigid avoidance of a mixture of 'brain-cells' and 'ideas' only applies to conceptual explanations, i.e. to the third step of the method of 'science.' There is no objection to conjoining both types in earlier stages where only a recording of a succession of phenomena is attempted, e.g. the statement that excessive ingestion of alcohol produces mental confusion. For a more detailed consideration of the nature of the physiological and psychological conceptions and of their relationship see the author's *Psychopathology* (Macmillan Company, 1927).

physiological and psychological conceptions bear to one another involves the much disputed question of the connection between mind and brain, and belongs to philosophy. It cannot of course, be entered upon here. From the point of view of science, a clear understanding of the simple distinction described above is all that is necessary.

An endeavour has been made to arrange the subject-matter of the book in such a way that the three successive steps of the method of science will appear in their logical order. Chapter III describes the phenomena of mental disorder, the facts which we observe in our patients. In chapter IV these facts are collected into groups, arranged, and classified. We then proceed in chapter V and other subsequent chapters to the *explanation* of these facts, the various psychological laws which resume the phenomena observed. The reader is here introduced to conceptual psychology, and his understanding of this difficult portion of the subject will be considerably clearer if he has adequately grasped the distinction between the phenomenal and conceptual outlined above. He will find that, in modern psychology, conceptions are employed which cannot be demonstrated to have an actual phenomenal existence. 'Complexes' and 'repression', for example, are conceptions devised to explain the phenomena which are observed, just as in physical science the concepts of 'force' and 'energy' are devised to explain the phenomena of motion. He will find, again, such conceptual abstractions as 'unconscious mental processes', involving the assumption that mental processes exist of which the individual himself is absolutely unconscious. It will perhaps appear at first sight that the assumption involves a psychological impossibility, and that if a mental process exists it must, *ipso facto*, be accompanied by consciousness. The reader must remember, however, that he is dealing with a conception which lays no claim to phenomenal reality, and that it belongs to the same generic type as the ether of the physicist.[1] An unconscious mental process is a phenomenal

[1] The view that unconscious mental processes are conceptual constructions is not accepted by the psychoanalytical school. This school maintains that

26

impossibility just as the weightless frictionless ether is a phenomenal impossibility. In both cases the conception justifies its claim to rank as a scientific theory, because it serves to resume and explain in a comprehensive and convenient manner the facts of our experience, and because it satisfies the one great criterion of science, the test of utility.

unconscious mental processes are inferred in the same way that the conscious processes of others are inferred and hence possess the same claim to phenomenal reality. For a fuller discussion of this point see *Psychopathology* (Macmillan Company, 1927), pp. 57 ff.

CHAPTER III

THE PHENOMENA OF MENTAL DISORDER

THE task which lies before us is to explain how the psychological conception may be applied to the phenomena of mental disorder, and to show that those phenomena are the result of definite psychological causes operating in accordance with definite psychological laws.

At the outset we encounter an obstacle which, though not perhaps peculiar to the subject we have chosen, offers exceptional difficulties on account of the conditions under which the subject has to be presented. We have to assume that our readers are ignorant, not only of the laws which govern the phenomena of mental disorder, but to a considerable extent of those phenomena themselves. Most readers will have some acquaintance with symptoms occurring in the minor forms of mental disorder known as 'neuroses', but few laymen have any practical experience of those occurring in the more pronounced forms of mental disorder included under 'insanity'. The conception of the insane patient possessed by the public at large is exaggerated and inaccurate. Hence before we can proceed to the explanation of the symptoms which the insane patient exhibits, it is necessary that this erroneous conception should be corrected, and we must ensure that our readers have at any rate a superficial acquaintance with the phenomena which actually occur. It is to this preliminary task that the present chapter is devoted.

To describe in a complete and systematic manner the symptoms met with in the manifold varieties of insanity is obviously impossible within the limits of a small book. We must be content to concentrate our attention upon a certain number of the more prominent manifestations which are apparent to any observer who visits the wards of a mental hospital. Our description will be far from exhaustive, and but little attempt will be made to achieve order or systematic grouping. The result will probably be comparable to the confused impression which the visitor we have imagined will carry away with him, but it will suffice to acquaint the reader with some of the actual facts of insanity, and with the technical terms which are employed to describe them. It is hoped, moreover, that this confused impression will be gradually removed in later chapters, and replaced by a more orderly picture in which each symptom will acquire its proper setting.

We shall commence with the description of certain general changes which may be regarded as affecting the mind as a whole, and then proceed to the enumeration of individual symptoms, selected either on account of the frequency of their occurrence, or because of their peculiarly striking character. It must be clearly understood that the phenomena we shall describe are in no sense mutually exclusive, and that many of them may occur together in one and the same case.

The first of the general changes we shall describe consists in a quantitative mental defect, a diminution in the general mental capacity involving all the functions of the mind. The patient cannot think, act, or remember efficiently, his intelligence is markedly below the average, and he seems abnormally stupid. This quantitative defect occurs in two forms, the congenital and the acquired, which are known respectively as *mental deficiency* and *dementia*.

In mental deficiency the patient is born without a normal mental equipment, and the mental powers never attain their full development. This failure of development may be of all possible grades, ranging from an almost complete absence of the mind to conditions in which intelligence is only slightly below the average. Patients of the lowest grades never progress beyond the mental status of an infant, they are incapable of speech or of the simplest adaptation to their environment, and require all their lives the care and attention customarily devoted to a baby. Others acquire speech, but cannot learn to read or write. Others, again, develop beyond this stage, but their knowledge remains very elementary, they never acquire any general ideas, and they are incapable of earning a living wage or of taking their place as citizens. Mental deficiency is generally correlated with an easily demonstrable failure of brain development.

In dementia the general defect of mental capacity is acquired. The patients have at one time possessed a normal mental equipment, but this has undergone a process of decay. The prototype of this process is the gradual failure of intelligence which occurs in normal old age, and some of the best examples of dementia may be seen in those cases where the mental decay of old age attains an extreme grade. Such cases are termed *senile dementia*, and are well described in Shakespeare's lines:

> Last scene of all,
> That ends this strange eventful history,
> Is second childishness and mere oblivion,
> Sans teeth, sans eyes, sans taste, sans everything.

But a similar quantitative loss may occur at any age, and may be of any degree, ranging from a simple blunting of mental acuity to a profound dementia in which the patient is incapable of the simplest mental operation. These acquired dementias are, like mental deficiency, generally correlated with marked changes in the brain.

In another variety of general mental change observed in cases of insanity, the alteration is qualitative rather than quantitative. It may be regarded as a change in the general attitude of the mind towards its experience, either transitory or more or less permanent. Under this heading are included *excitement*, *depression*, and *apathy*.

Everyone is acquainted with the meaning of excitement, and the term does not require further definition. It is a symptom of frequent occurrence in insanity, where it differs from the similar phenomenon met with in normal mental life mainly in the exaggeration of its manifestation, in the apparent lack of an adequate cause, and in the fact that it is out of harmony with the patient's real condition and circumstances. Excitement as a symptom of insanity appears in many forms, differing from one another in almost every feature, except in the fundamental fact that the mind is exhibiting an abnormal output of energy. One of the commonest forms is known as *manic* excitement, a variety which will be best illustrated by the description of an actual case.

The patient is in a state of constant activity, commencing a new occupation at every moment, and immediately abandoning it in favour of another. He is never still, but exhibits a continual *press of activity*. He talks rapidly and without intermission, flying from one subject to another, with but little logical connection. He seems incapable of carrying out any connected train of thought, his attention is caught by every trifling object, and as soon diverted again. He is, generally, abnormally cheerful and absurdly pleased with himself and his environment, though his mood is as mutable as his attention, and changes to anger at the smallest provocation.

Under certain circumstances we might be disposed to regard such behaviour as pardonable, though exaggerated and ill-balanced. When, however, we discover that the patient is emaciated and in wretched health, that he has recently undergone a series of terrible stresses, that the fortunes of himself and his family are at their lowest ebb, and that now the crowning misfortune of removal to a mental hospital has befallen him, then his present behaviour becomes altogether incomprehensible. It is so out of harmony with the actual facts of his position, that we have no hesitation in regarding his conduct as definitely insane.

In other varieties the excitement is more extreme, the cheerfulness is, perhaps, suddenly replaced by bouts of furious anger, the patient attacks all those about him, is altogether impervious to reason and to argument, and presents a picture approximating to the popular conception of the maniac.

Depression may be regarded as the converse of excitement. The patient is slow in all his actions, thinks with difficulty, and is miserable and unhappy.

In the third qualitative general change, *apathy*, the patient is neither excited nor depressed, but absolutely indifferent, and without apparent interests, desires, or ambitions. Apathy is best exemplified in the so-called *emotional dementia* which characterises many of the chronic patients who constitute the permanent population of the hospital. The patient sits in a corner of the ward with expressionless face and head hanging down, making no attempt to occupy himself in any way, evincing no interest in anything that goes on around him, and apparently noticing nothing. If we address him, we obtain no answer, or perhaps at the best a monosyllabic reply, often quite irrelevant to the question asked.

At first sight such a case would seem to present a genuine dementia, an actual quantitative loss of mental capacity of the type described earlier in this chapter. If, however, we succeed in obtaining an insight into the patient's mind, we find that the dementia is largely only apparent; the patient can observe, remember, and carry out complicated trains of thought, if only we can provide him with the necessary stimulus. The explanation of the condition lies in the profound emotional apathy present. The patient is completely inert, and makes no use of his mental faculties, because he has no interests or desires. The whole external world resembles for him those innumerable trivial things which we pass by without attention or notice at every moment of our lives—an object unworthy of the expenditure of any mental energy.

In the less pronounced forms of emotional dementia the patients will answer our questions, and perhaps carry out routine tasks with machine-like regularity. But they evince no interests, they have no hopes, plans, or ambitions, and they are content to remain permanently in the narrow world of the hospital.

In addition to the general changes so far described there occur in mental disorder a vast number of individual symptoms of the most varied kinds. We shall now proceed to enumerate some of these symptoms, selected in haphazard fashion, and without attempt at classification or coherent order.

The first symptom which we shall select for description is 'somnambulism'. This phenomenon, which is more commonly met with in those so-called 'neurotic' cases belonging to the ill-defined borderland between sanity and insanity, may be exemplified by an account of the case described by Prof. Janet under the name of 'Irène'.

Irène had nursed her mother through a prolonged illness culminating in death. The circumstances connected with the death were peculiarly painful, and the event produced a profound shock upon the patient's mind. An abnormal mental condition developed, characterised by the frequent appearance of symptoms resembling those exhibited by the ordinary sleep-walker. Irène, perhaps engaged at the moment in sewing or in conversation, would suddenly cease her occupation, and would commence to live over again the scene of her mother's death, carrying out every detail with all the power of an accomplished actress. While this drama was in progress she was perfectly unconscious of the actual events happening in her environment, heard nothing that was said to her, and saw nothing but the imaginary scene in which she was living at the moment. This phenomenon, technically termed a *somnambulism*, would end as suddenly as it had begun, and Irène would return to her former occupation, absolutely unaware of the fact that it had ever been interrupted. After an interval of perhaps several days a second somnambulism, resembling the first in all respects, would appear in the same abrupt manner. If the patient were interrogated during the apparently normal intervals it would be found not only that she had entirely forgotten everything which had happened during the somnambulism, but that the whole system of ideas connected with her mother's death had completely disappeared from her mind. She remembered nothing of the illness or its tragic end; discussed her mother without emotion, and was reproached by her relatives for her callous indifference to the whole subject. This curious localised loss of memory or *amnesia* will be more fully discussed in a subsequent chapter, when its precise nature and causation will be explained.

The next group of symptoms to which we may direct our attention comprises *hallucinations* and *delusions*. These phenomena occupy an important place amongst the manifestations of insanity, and may be observed in a large percentage of patients.

Hallucinations may be roughly defined as false sense-impressions. For example, the patient sees an object which has no real existence, or hears an imaginary voice. Hallucinations are termed visual, auditory, tactile, etc., according to the sense to which the false impression appears to belong. Auditory hallucinations are particularly common. The 'voices' may make remarks of either a pleasant or an unpleasant character, but generally they refer to subjects closely related to the patient's most intimate life, and often they consist of some abusive comment or reproach reiterated with stereotyped persistence. Thus a patient may hear a voice constantly announcing that on account of the sins he has committed he will shortly be put to death. Frequently, in order to explain these strange phenomena, the patient constructs some fantastic hypothesis, and persuades himself, for example, that they are produced by 'wireless telephones' or 'spiritualism'.

Delusions are closely allied to hallucinations, and generally accompany the latter. The distinction lies in the fact that delusions are not false sensations, but false beliefs. Thus if a patient sees an object which has no objective reality he has an hallucination, but if he believes that he is the Emperor of the World he has a delusion. Delusions may be of all kinds, but there are two groups which call for special mention on account of their great frequency, *grandiose* and *persecutory*. In the former the patient believes himself to be some exalted personage, or to possess some other attribute which raises him far above the level of his fellows. He may believe, for example, that he is the king, or a millionaire, or a great inventor. In some cases no actual delusions are expressed, but the exaggerated sense of self-importance is betrayed by affectations of gait and manner, by the employment of a fantastically pedantic phraseology, or by other similar manifestations.

A patient who exhibits the second, or persecutory, type of delusion believes that deliberate attempts are made to harm him in some way. Thus he may believe that certain people are plotting to destroy his life. Both grandiose and persecutory delusions are often associated with hallucinations; voices hail the patient as the rightful owner of the throne, or cover him with abuse and threaten some dire fate. The two types are frequently combined; for example, a patient may maintain that he is the king, but that an organised conspiracy exists to deprive him of his birthright. In this way delusions are sometimes elaborated into an extraordinarily complicated system, and every fact of the patient's experience is distorted until it is capable of taking its place in the delusional scheme.

An important variety of persecutory false belief is constituted by the so-called 'delusions of reference'. The patient misconstrues every event which happens in his environment, however trivial it may be, believes that it is directly bound up with his fate, and that it is in some way designed to injure him. If he observes two of his fellows talking together he immediately assumes that he is the subject of their conversation, and every accidental misfortune is regarded as a deliberate attempt to annoy him. Sometimes this misconstruction is carried to lengths which are fantastically absurd; a trifling displacement of the furniture of the patient's room is thought to be a signal employed by his enemies, and a spot upon his dinner plate is proof positive that poison is being introduced into his food.

The most striking feature of a delusion is its fixity and imperviousness to all opposing argument. Persuasion and reason are altogether ineffectual against it, and the patient preserves his belief in spite of the most convincing demonstration of its falsity.

The extent to which conduct is affected by the presence of delusions is, however, very variable. In some cases patients under the influence of persecutory ideas will commit serious assaults upon their imagined enemies, and become a source of great danger to the community. In a very large number of cases, on the other hand, the delusion seems to have no direct

35

effect upon the patient's behaviour. Often, indeed, belief and conduct are completely divorced from one another, or even grotesquely inconsistent. Thus, the 'Queen of the World' will contentedly carry out her daily task of scrubbing the ward floor, and the omnipotent millionaire will beg plaintively for a small gift of tobacco.

We may next proceed to consider the group of phenomena included under the term *obsession*, which bear a close superficial resemblance to delusions, but must be carefully distinguished therefrom. Obsessions, indeed, rarely occur in actual insanity, but are a characteristic feature of certain types of neurotic disorder. An obsession may be defined as the 'overweighting' of a particular element in consciousness. The patient complains of some idea which constantly recurs to his mind in spite of all efforts to banish it, or he is constantly impelled to carry out some irrelevant and inappropriate action. For example, he is haunted by the idea that he is suffering from cancer; he is perfectly aware that no foundation for this suspicion exists, and that no symptom of the dreaded disease is actually present. He does not, in fact, really *believe* that he has cancer, but he cannot banish the idea from his mind, and he needs constantly to reassure himself of its erroneous character. It is this absence of a definite false belief that constitutes the essential distinction between an obsession and a delusion.

Or, again, the patient is impelled to carry out repeatedly some needless and useless action. Thus Freud describes the case of a lady who had an overwhelming need to examine in the most careful manner the number of every bank-note which came into her possession. A not uncommon variety of obsession is the so-called 'washing mania', in which the patient is driven to wash his hands at almost every moment of the day. He fully realises the absurdity of this performance, but the compulsion is irresistible, and all his available time and energy are squandered in a fruitless struggle to combat the obsession.

We may next direct our attention to a curious phenomenon most frequently observed in chronic cases of insanity of long duration, the 'stereotyped action'. The patient carries out some action with monotonous repetition and regularity day in and day out. Often all his mental energy is absorbed in this performance, so that from one year's end to another he seems to have no other interest, desire, or ambition. These stereotyped actions may be of all kinds, and of all degrees of complexity, ranging from a simple rhythmical movement of the hands or head to elaborate procedures suggesting the manipulations of a skilled tradesman who is plying his craft. Sometimes, again, a phrase or sentence is repeated over and over with the same monotonous persistence. Thus, one of my patients has for years devoted his entire waking existence to reciting the phrase, 'It's all wrong, I tell you.'

Alterations in speech and phraseology form an important part of the symptomatology of insanity. The rapid flow of disconnected talk occurring in manic excitement has already been mentioned. Often, however, the changes observed are much more profound. The phrases are curiously distorted, individual words are displaced or omitted, all grammatical form seems to be lost, and the patient's whole conversation is an incoherent and meaningless hotch-potch. The following is an excellent example of such incoherent speech: 'What spelling letters have you there, do you write it in Greek, do you write strength, that photography is trouble, ex parte, posse comitatis, I get that, Mr John McCall's stereotypist, physiological design, that's the result on the blue line, it comes up to you on the strength of duty . . . .'

Sometimes an exaggeratedly pedantic phraseology is employed, in which polysyllabic words are often employed without any regard to their precise meaning. One patient complains, for example, that his health has been 'deflected', and that he is the victim of 'illegal circumstances and cruel conventions'. It will be seen later that such pedantic phraseology is generally employed to emphasise the importance of the patient or of the statements which he is making, and we have already observed that it is closely allied to the grandiose delusions and affectations of gait and manner dealt with above.

37

This cursory description of some of the symptoms met with in insanity must suffice for the present. Its imperfections have already been pointed out, and we can hardly hope that the reader will have obtained from it that clear picture of insanity which practical acquaintance with patients can alone give. Other symptoms, however, will be described in the course of subsequent chapters as occasion arises, and the more complete accounts of individual cases to be found therein will give a better understanding of the way in which the various phenomena are combined together, and of their mode of development.

CHAPTER IV

DISSOCIATION

In the preceding chapter we have collected together certain of the more prominent phenomena of mental disorder. To the uninitiated eye they appear as a chaos of disconnected facts, each seemingly independent of all the rest. A careful examination will show, however, that there are certain general attributes common to many of the symptoms displayed by our patients. With the aid of these general attributes it is possible to classify the phenomena into groups, and thereby to reduce the confusion to some sort of order.

Firstly, the conditions described as mental deficiency and dementia may be placed in a separate group. They depend, as we have seen, upon an absolute quantitative defect of mental capacity, and are in this respect fundamentally different from all the other phenomena dealt with in chapter III. These conditions are generally accompanied by a correlated defect in the structure of the brain, and it must be frankly confessed that, in the present state of knowledge, the psychological conception is of relatively little value in the study of their causation, and that the physiological conception is a far more profitable instrument of investigation. It is true, of course, that psychology is compelled to take account of such quantitative defects of mental capacity, and that it is able to explain the relation which they bear to many of the other phenomena of insanity, but the questions involved are complicated and difficult, and cannot be satisfactorily considered without presupposing a considerable practical acquaintance with the subject. We shall therefore make no attempt to deal further with mental deficiency and dementia in this book, but devote all our attention to the qualitative changes in mental function forming the bulk of the phenomena described in the preceding chapter.

We shall at once observe that many of these symptoms are

only exaggerated forms of mental processes with which we are all acquainted. The symptoms described as excitement and depression, for example, differ from the similar conditions seen in normal men only by their intensity and by their seeming lack of any adequate cause. Similarly, the affective disturbance referred to as 'emotional dementia' is but an exaggeration of the apathy and lack of volition so frequently met with in everyday life.

Other of the affective symptoms, however, seem to be further removed from the normal—the emotions are not only exaggerated, but distorted and senseless. Similarly the incoherent, apparently meaningless phrases exhibited by some of our patients have but little obvious relation to the language and thought which we find in ourselves. Finally, we meet with symptoms which seem altogether strange and incomprehensible—hallucinations and delusions, for example. Here our analogies fail us altogether, and we are tempted to limit our explanation to the simple statement that the man is mad, and that is all there is to say about the matter.

> to define true madness,
> What is't but to be nothing else but mad.

Yet we shall find as we proceed that even the most bizarre symptoms are not so very different from processes to be discovered in our own minds, and that the insane patient appears more and more like ourselves the better we are enabled to penetrate into the tortuous recesses of his spirit.

In order that the reader may acquire some of this understanding, it is necessary that he should be first introduced to a conception which plays an important part throughout the whole of abnormal psychology, that of 'dissociation of consciousness'.

If we are asked to turn our mental eye inwards and carefully observe at any given moment the content of our mind—or, as it is technically termed, the momentary 'field of consciousness' —we should probably describe it as an indivisible whole, a uniform stream of thought progressing towards some definite end. It would not appear to be composed of separate parts, each proceeding independently of the others, but of sensations, ideas, and volitions all united in some common aim. If I am engaged upon a mathematical problem, then my field of consciousness seems to consist at the moment solely of the various mental processes necessary to the solution of the problem. A few moments later my attention may perhaps be diverted to making plans for a forthcoming holiday, but the mathematical problem will then have temporarily retired from the field of consciousness; the problem and the holiday plans do not both occupy the mind at once, although our attention may rapidly oscillate from one to the other. We should find, moreover, that in spite of the fact that mathematics and holidays have apparently nothing in common, there was nevertheless some link which carried my mind over the gap between them, and that in reality no break in the continuity of the stream of thought occurred.

Yet this statement is only partially true of the normal mind, and it is hardly true at all in the case of some of our patients. Their minds are frequently very far from being uniform streams of thought, progressing towards some definite end, but are on the contrary composed of more or less isolated mental processes, each pursuing its own development. This division of the mind into independent fragments, which are not co-ordinated together to attain some common end, is termed 'dissociation of consciousness'. A few examples of various degrees of dissociation will make our meaning clear.

It has been pointed out that even the normal mind does not always present that undivided field of consciousness which we might be tempted at first sight to ascribe to it. Suppose, for example, I sit at the piano and play a piece of music. If I am a sufficiently expert performer it is possible that I may at the same time be able to carry on a complex train of independent thought, let us say the solution of some problem of conduct. My mind does not under these circumstances present a uniform field of consciousness, but one divided into two parts or processes. Each of these processes requires a considerable expenditure of mental energy. The piece of music is perhaps one which I have never seen before, and it has to be played with appropriate and constantly varying expression—while the problem of conduct may be similarly complicated in its character. Each of these activities is almost entirely independent of the other, yet both can be carried on at the same moment. The field of consciousness must therefore be divided into two portions, in other words a certain degree of dissociation of consciousness must be present. Similar remarks apply to many other simultaneous activities; for example, those exhibited by the skilled tradesman who plies his craft while his mind is at the same time occupied with other matters.

In all these cases, however, the dissociation of consciousness is temporary, and only partial in character. Both activities are under the control of the subject, and either may be abandoned at will. In the more marked degrees of dissociation found in our patients this control no longer exists.

Let us take, for example, the phenomenon of 'automatic writing'. This curious condition, although occasionally exhibited by comparatively normal people, attains its most perfect development in the form of disorder known as hysteria. Suppose that we engage an hysterical patient in conversation and, while his attention is thus diverted, insert a pencil between the fingers of his right hand. If a third person now whispers some question into the patient's ear, it may be possible to induce him to write answers to those questions, although he continues all the time to discuss with us some totally different subject. Under such circumstances it will be found that the patient is entirely unconscious of what his hand is doing, and is, moreover, often altogether ignorant of the events which the writing describes. These events frequently relate to episodes in the patient's past life which he appears to have completely forgotten, and the experiment is occasionally employed with the object of resuscitating such buried memories. It may be remarked that this loss of memory for some definite section of the patient's past experience, often extending over a considerable period of time and including events of great importance, is a characteristic symptom of hysteria.

Automatic writing has played a large part in the history of spiritualism, and has been attributed by supporters of that doctrine to the activity of some spiritual being who avails himself of the patient's hand in order to manifest to the world his desires and opinions. So far as the phenomenon itself is concerned, however, the explanation is comparatively simple. A dissociation has taken place, though one far more complete than those hitherto described. The field of consciousness is divided into two distinct parts, one engaged in conversation, the other comprising the systems of ideas which are finding expression in the automatic writing. Each portion carries on complicated mental processes, and yet each is not only independent of the other, but totally unaware of that other's existence. The patient's mind seems, in fact, to be split into two smaller minds, engaged in two different occupations, making use of two distinct sets of memories, and without any relations whatever one to the other. Such a case, therefore, provides us with a perfect example of dissociation of consciousness. But it must always be remembered that, however strange and incomprehensible such advanced dissociations may at first sight seem to be, yet they are nothing but exaggerated forms of those dissociations which have been seen to occur in every normal individual.

Let us now proceed to the consideration of a type of dissociation only slightly different from that just described. We found that in the uniform stream of thought characteristic of the normal mind there was no break or gap in the continuity of ideas. However abruptly a new idea might arise in consciousness, yet it was always possible to demonstrate that the apparent gap was really bridged by some associative link. The consciousness of any given moment, moreover, was always perfectly aware of the mental processes which had taken place in the consciousness of the preceding moment. Now it is possible to imagine that this continuity in the stream of consciousness should suddenly cease to exist, that the stream should be, as it were, suddenly broken across. The content of consciousness immediately after the break would then be absolutely independent of the content of consciousness in the moment preceding the break. All relations between the two would be severed, and the consciousness of the second moment would therefore be entirely unaware of what had been contained in the consciousness of the first moment. The mind of the individual would, in fact, suddenly be filled with a new series of ideas, while it would at the same time be altogether ignorant of the ideas which had occupied it a moment previously. We have here, not a dissociation of consciousness into two separate simultaneously present portions, but a dissociation of the consciousness of one moment from the consciousness which preceded it. This is the type of dissociation which occurs in somnambulism. In the case of Irène, described in the last chapter (p. 33), we saw that at the onset of a somnambulism the train of thought occupying the patient's mind was abruptly broken off and replaced by an entirely different set of ideas. Whatever she had previously been engaged upon, the beginning of the somnambulism was characterised by the sudden invasion into consciousness of the ideas and memories connected with her mother's death. She would live through the deathbed scene again and again, her whole mind absorbed in the phantasy, and altogether oblivious of what was actually taking place around her. Then suddenly the somnambulism would cease, and she would 'return to herself'. In other words, the train of ideas constituting the somnambulism would abruptly disappear from consciousness, and would be replaced, equally abruptly, by the ideas and actions which had occupied her mind at the moment when the somnambulism commenced. If the patient, after this 'return to herself', were questioned concerning her recent doings, she would be found to be absolutely ignorant of everything which had taken place during the somnambulism. Her memory would show a gap extending from the exact moment when the somnambulism began to the exact moment when it ceased. We should find, in fact, that the continuous stream of her thought had been interrupted by the sudden appearance of a 'dissociated system of ideas', which occupied the entire field of consciousness for a certain time, and then as suddenly disappeared. In such a case the continuity of transition observed in the normal mind has been replaced by an abrupt change from one train of ideas to another train which has no relation to the first. If we compare the field of consciousness to a cinematograph screen, then the normal process corresponds to the continuous change in the picture produced by a single film, while the dissociated processes occurring in somnambulism correspond to the effect obtained by abruptly breaking off one film, and replacing it by another representing an altogether different subject. The type of dissociation seen in automatic writing, on the other hand, would be produced by employing two films at the same moment, each projecting its picture upon a separate portion of the same screen.

The dissociated system of ideas whose eruption into the field of consciousness is responsible for the appearance of a somnambulism, may attain to any degree of complexity and development. In the case of Irène its structure was relatively simple, and it comprised but little beyond the ideas connected with the mother's illness and death. Hence, while the somnambulism was in progress, the patient's mental life seemed narrowed down to the expression of those ideas; she was totally insusceptible to all other impressions, and incapable of adapting herself to the actual conditions of her environment. In some cases, however, the dissociated system is far more extensive and more completely developed, including within itself whole tracts of the patient's mental life. Under these circumstances the patient's behaviour may be comparatively normal, and adapted to the environment, even when the dissociated system is in entire possession of the field. Such cases are not generally termed somnambulisms, although they are precisely similar to the latter in their fundamental characters, but are regarded as examples of 'double personality'.

Double personality is a phenomenon which has aroused considerable popular interest, owing, no doubt, to the dramatic character of its manifestations. It has furnished fascinating material for works of fiction, headed by the famous 'Dr Jekyll and Mr Hyde' of R. L. Stevenson. A large number of actual cases, however, have now been described, and in its less perfect forms double personality is by no means so rare as is generally supposed. As an illustrative example we may quote the case of the Rev. Ansel Bourne, originally described by William James.

On 17 January 1887, the Rev. Ansel Bourne, an itinerant preacher, drew a considerable sum of money from a bank in Providence, and then entered a tram-car. This was the last incident which he remembered.

He did not return home that day, and nothing was heard of him for two months. . . . On the morning of 14 March, however, at Norristown, Pennsylvania, a man calling himself A. J. Brown, who had rented a small shop six weeks previously, stocked it with stationery, confectionery, fruit and small articles, and carried on his quiet trade without seeming to anyone unnatural or eccentric, woke up in a fright and called in the people of the house to tell him where he was. He said that his name was Ansel Bourne, that he knew nothing of shopkeeping, and that the last thing he remembered—it seemed only yesterday—was drawing the money from the bank in Providence.

Now it will at once be apparent that in this case an extensive dissociation had occurred. The normal stream of consciousness was suddenly broken across and replaced by a series of altogether different mental processes. This new system, sufficiently complex in its structure to permit of the patient leading an orderly existence, occupied the stage for two months, when it disappeared with equal abruptness and the former stream resumed its course. It will be clear that such a case differs from a somnambulism only in the more elaborate development of the systems of ideas concerned.

All the examples of dissociation so far given show us systems of ideas, or trains of thought, which are split off from the rest of consciousness, and which lead an independent existence.

Let us now examine these examples more closely, with a view to determining what exactly we are to understand by this 'splitting off' of a system of ideas. In both automatic writing and somnambulism two well-marked characters are present. Firstly, the main body of consciousness—or, as it is usually termed, the personality or *ego*—has no knowledge of the dissociated system. Thus Irène in her normal state had no memory of the actions and ideas which had filled the period of somnambulism. Secondly, the dissociated system develops autonomously, that is to say it pursues its own course without any dependence upon the main body of consciousness. It is, in fact, altogether exempt from the control of the personality. Irène could not decide beforehand what actions should be carried out in her somnambulisms. The ideas connected with her mother's death developed as a self-contained system, over which the personality could exercise no influence whatever.

The same characters distinguish the phenomenon of automatic writing. Firstly, the patient is quite unaware of what his hand is writing, or even of the fact that it is in movement. Secondly, the personality has no power to direct what the hand shall write, or to alter in any way the train of ideas which it is expressing.

The question now arises whether both the characters described are to be regarded as the essential marks of a dissociated or 'split off' system of ideas, or whether we may speak of dissociation when only one of these characters is present; and if only one need be present, which is to be regarded as essential—the fact that the personality is unaware of the existence of the dissociated system, or the fact that the latter develops independently and is exempt from the control of the former.

Now a little consideration will show that all cases which exhibit the first character must inevitably exhibit the second also. If the mind of a certain patient contains a system of ideas of which the personality is absolutely ignorant, then that system must obviously be independent, and exempt from the control of the personality. The first character, therefore, presupposes the second. It is, in fact, only an extreme degree of the second. All cases which display it possess not only a separated, independent, and autonomous system of ideas, but one of whose existence the personality is in addition unaware. We therefore reach the conclusion that 'unawareness' is only a special example of 'independence', and hence that 'independence' is the more fundamental and comprehensive character. It will be found convenient to make the term 'dissociation' indicate only this fundamental character of independence, and to regard unawareness on the part of the personality merely as a special case of dissociation. We may express this position by the following definition: A system of ideas is said to be dissociated when it is divorced from the personality, and when its course and development are exempt from the control of the personality.

We are now in a position to proceed further in the examination of our patients, and to determine if there are not other symptoms than automatic writing, somnambulism, and double personality, which may be brought under this definition of dissociation. Consider, for example, the case of obsessions. If we inquire of the patient mentioned on p. 36, why she so conscientiously studies the number of every bank-note which comes into her possession, she replies, 'I do not know why I do so, but I simply cannot help it. Whenever I see a bank-note, something forces me to examine the number. Of course I am distressed at my foolish behaviour, but the impulse is absolutely uncontrollable.' In other words, the sight of a bank-note arouses a system of ideas, whose development the patient's personality is altogether unable to control. Whatever she may herself desire to do, this system will pursue its course until it has achieved its end, and she will be compelled to look at the number. She is, of course, perfectly aware of her action, but cannot alter it or prevent it. We have here a system of ideas which is separate from, and develops independently of, the personality, and which our definition therefore entitles us to describe as dissociated. This type of dissociation differs from that seen in automatic writing in the fact that the personality is aware of the existence of the dissociated system. The independence of the dissociated system is, however, equally evident in both.

Similar remarks hold good of the various other obsessive actions, e.g. 'washing mania', which we have observed in certain of our patients.

It should be remarked that phenomena analogous to these latter symptoms frequently occur in the experience of every normal individual. For example, the melody which 'runs in one's head' continuously, and will not be banished; the absurd and irrelevant idea which insistently recurs to one's mind in defiance of all the laws of logic; the irresistible impulse to touch every lamp-post one passes, and so on. In all these cases, just as in those more exaggerated instances which occur in our patients, we have dissociated fragments of mind which pursue their own course without relation to the conscious aims and desires of the personality. The personality is aware of the existence of the dissociated system, but is aware of it as something outside of and foreign to itself. As the patient will frequently express it—'the idea forces itself into my mind', 'something suddenly compels me to do this action'.

These obsessional cases, in which the dissociated system appears to the personality as a foreign body which has intruded itself into the mind, serve as a bridge to carry us over to yet another type of dissociation. Consider the cases described in the last chapter in which hallucinations of various kinds occur. We found, for example, a patient who constantly heard voices announcing that on account of the sins he had committed he would shortly be put to death. Now we know that these voices did not correspond to any actual reality in the external world. Although to the patient himself they seemed intensely real, to the bystander they were nothing but figments of the imagination. In other words, they existed only in the patient's mind, and were, in fact, merely a portion of his own consciousness. But, although the voices formed a part of the mind, yet it is obvious that they did not form a part of the personality. It will hence be evident that the voices, and the system of ideas which the voices express, are to be regarded as dissociated portions of the patient's own consciousness. Strictly speaking, it would be better to say that the system of ideas in question is dissociated from the personality, and that the hallucinatory 'voice' is the mode in which the dissociated system announces its existence to the personality. This splitting of the patient's consciousness into two parts, one of which talks to the other, is a frequent phenomenon in every mental hospital.

The conception of dissociation enables us, again, to represent more clearly to ourselves the mental state of the patient who possesses a delusion. A delusion, it will be remembered, is a false belief which is impervious to the most complete logical demonstration of its impossibility, and unshaken by the presence of incompatible or obviously contradictory facts. Thus, if a patient believes that he is the king, it is useless to prove conclusively to him that his contention is wrong; he remains serenely unaffected. He is, perhaps, well acquainted with the past history of himself and his family, but it never occurs to him that the facts contained therein are incompatible with the belief that he is the son of George III. He may assure us that he is omnipotent and capable of creating a new universe, and yet the next moment he may ask plaintively to be allowed to leave the hospital, or beg for a small quantity of tobacco. This tissue of contradictions seems at first sight inexplicable and incomprehensible, but the key to the riddle is clear so soon as we realise that the patient's mind is in a state of dissociation. It no longer presents a homogeneous stream progressing in a definite direction towards a single end, but is composed of more or less isolated mental processes, each pursuing its own independent development, unaffected by the presence of its fellows. The patient believes that he is the king, and he is also aware of facts which totally contradict that belief; but although both these things exist together in his mind, they are not allowed to come into contact, and each is impervious to the significance of the other. They pursue their courses in logic-tight compartments, as it were, separated by barriers through which no connecting thought or reasoning is permitted to pass. Similarly, the patient's belief is unaffected by our scientific demonstration of its impossibility. He understands perfectly each point of our reasoning, but its significance is not allowed to penetrate the compartment which contains his delusion; it glides off as water glides off a duck's back.

Although the phenomena just described are so bizarre, and so characteristically insane, yet this dissociation of the mind into logic-tight compartments is by no means confined to the population of the mental hospital. It is a common, and perhaps inevitable, occurrence in the psychology of every human being. Our political convictions are notoriously inaccessible to argument, and we preserve the traditional beliefs of our childhood in spite of the contradictory facts constantly presented by our experience. Such phenomena can only be explained by the existence of a certain amount of dissociation, and, though less in degree, it is precisely similar in kind to the dissociation which permits the asylum queen to scrub the ward floor, serenely unconscious of the incongruity between her exalted rank and her menial occupation.

CHAPTER V

COMPLEXES

In chapter III we have described some of the phenomena to be observed in various morbid states of mind, and in chapter IV we have endeavoured to arrange these phenomena into groups. This process of classification has enabled us to reduce the original chaos into some sort of order, and to obtain a comprehensive view of the facts of our subject. We have discovered, for example, that many of the manifestations of mental disorder are to be regarded as cases of dissociation of consciousness—the stream of consciousness is divided into independent currents no longer combined into one harmonious whole. So far, however, no attempt has been made to explain why these phenomena occur. We have seen that the imaginary voices which torture the hallucinated patient are nothing but split-off portions of his own consciousness, but we have assigned no reason to account for a portion of consciousness being split off in this abnormal manner, nor have we explained why the hallucinatory voice should make remarks of one character rather than another. We have found, in fact, that certain events occur, but we are still altogether in the dark as to why they occur.

The reader who has clearly understood the general principles enunciated in chapter II will at once perceive that we have carried out the first two steps of the method of science, but have as yet made no attempt to proceed to the third step. The phenomena have been collected and classified; we have still to find conceptions which will suffice to resume and explain those phenomena.

This necessary third step is one of great difficulty. The science of psychiatry is so young, so much remains to be discovered, that it is only possible at the present day to advance a short distance in the desired direction. Moreover, even this short distance will inevitably take us into disputed ground, for the frontier of a youthful science is always the scene of constant battle. Hence, although the clear presentation of our subject will necessitate the adoption of a somewhat dogmatic attitude, the reader must remember that many of the conclusions reached in this and the following chapters are to be regarded as tentative rather than as firmly established. To a large extent they are the result of the researches carried out in recent years by Prof. Freud of Vienna and Dr Jung of Zürich.

Before we endeavour to discover the causes underlying morbid psychological phenomena we must be convinced that our quest is reasonable, we must firmly believe that such causes exist. This belief involves the adoption of psychological determinism—the doctrine that in the psychical world, as in the world of matter, every event must have a cause. Provided that the necessary antecedents are present, then the result will inevitably follow; and if we see the result, then we know that certain definite causes must have combined in order to produce it. Chance has no more part in psychology than it has in physics. Every thought which flits through the mind, however casual or irrelevant it may seem to be, is the only thought which can possibly result from the various mental processes which preceded it. If I am asked to think of a number, it is apparently a matter of indifference to me which number I select. In reality, however, the number is definitely and absolutely determined by the mental state of the moment— one particular number will inevitably appear in the mind, no other is possible. This position will perhaps strike the reader as strained and unreal, but unless it is adopted as a preliminary axiom, no science of psychology can exist. Whatever our private philosophy may be, so long as we are thinking psychologically and scientifically, we must subscribe to all the implications of the law of causation.

The ascertaining of the causes determining the flow of our consciousness is the ultimate aim of psychology. We shall expect, of course, that the laws discovered will be identical in the sane and the insane, just as the physiological laws

C

determining the processes of the diseased body are the same as those determining the processes of the healthy body—the difference is merely one of degree and combination in the causes concerned.

Now we may get an idea of the direction in which we should search for these determinative causes by the consideration of some simple examples. Let us suppose that I am an enthusiastic photographer. It is obvious that the existence of this hobby will continually affect the flow of my consciousness. Scenes which would otherwise be indifferent to me will frequently arouse interest as possible material for a picture: if I peruse a newspaper an article upon photography will at once arrest my attention, and when I meet my friends I shall probably seize every opportunity to turn the conversation to my favourite pursuit. We see, in fact, that the hobby is one of the causes determining the direction of my thinking. Now, if we endeavour to ascertain the exact nature of a hobby, we find that it is a system of connected ideas, with a strong emotional tone, and a tendency to produce actions of a certain definite character. Such a system of emotionally toned ideas is termed in technical language a 'complex'—and a hobby is to be regarded as a particular variety of complex. In the simple case just described we should say that one of the causes determining the flow of my consciousness was a strong 'photography complex'.[1]

Complexes may be of all sorts and kinds, the component ideas may be of every variety, the accompanying emotional tones pleasant or painful, very intense or comparatively weak.

When the emotional tone of a complex is very intense, the action which it exerts upon consciousness becomes correspondingly great. Consider, for example, the immensely powerful complex formed in the young man who has recently fallen in

[1] The term 'complex' was originally devised by Jung, and used by him in the general sense employed in this book. Its connotation has tended to become restricted, however, to systems of ideas which are repressed (see chapter VII), and therefore of a more or less morbid character. The more general conception employed in the present chapter corresponds closely to the 'sentiment' of Shand and McDougall.

love. Ideas belonging to the complex incessantly emerge into consciousness, the slightest associative connections sufficing to arouse them. All his mental energy is absorbed in weaving trains of thought centred in the beloved one, and he cannot divert his mind to the business of the day. Every event which happens is brought into relation with his passion, and the whole universe is for him nothing but a setting for his dominating complex.

Complexes, then, are causes which determine the behaviour of the conscious stream, and the action which they exert upon consciousness may be regarded as the psychological analogue of the conception of 'force' in physics. They are not, of course, constantly active, but only become so under certain conditions. These conditions consist in the presence of a 'stimulus', occurring whenever one or more of the ideas belonging to a complex is roused to activity, either by some external event, or by processes of association occurring within the mind itself. Thus, in the simple example we have taken the 'photography complex' might be stimulated by a conversation in which some photographic subject was introduced, or by a chain of associations leading from some indifferent idea to an idea definitely belonging to the sphere of photography. So soon as this necessary stimulation has occurred, the complex immediately tends to exert its effect upon consciousness. The effect consists normally in the introduction into consciousness of ideas, emotions, and trains of activity belonging to the complex. Of the ideas, arguments, etc., presented to the individual, those which are in harmony with the complex are reinforced, whereas those not so in harmony tend to be inhibited and to lose their cogency.

The mode of thought produced in this manner by the activity of a complex is quite different from that occurring in genuine logical thinking. In the latter case each step is the logical consequence of the preceding steps, evidence is impartially weighed, and the probability of various solutions is dispassionately considered. Such genuine logical thinking is in ordinary life comparatively rare; in most cases a 'complex bias' is only too obvious. Even in the world of science, generally regarded by the ignorant as the peculiar sphere of dispassionate and cold thought, complexes play a vast part. The discussions of any learned society provide most instructive material in this respect.

In these systems of emotionally toned ideas we have therefore found efficient causes which are at any rate partially responsible for the direction of our thoughts and actions. We may now proceed a stage further. If we asked the photographer why he always thought and acted in certain ways he would probably at once reply, 'Because I am interested in photography'; that is to say, he would himself be aware of the existence of the photography-complex and of the way in which it produced its effects. This subjective awareness of the existence and action of a complex is, however, by no means always present. A complex may exert a pronounced effect upon consciousness, although the individual himself may be unaware of its action—that is to say, he may be altogether ignorant of the causes which are really determining his own mental processes. An example will help to make this statement intelligible. When a party politician is called upon to consider a new measure, his verdict is largely determined by certain constant systems of ideas and trends of thought, constituting what is generally known as 'party bias'. We should describe these systems in our newly acquired terminology as his 'political-complex'. The complex causes him to take up an attitude towards the proposed measure which is quite independent of any absolute merits that the latter may possess. If we argue with our politician, we shall find that the complex will reinforce in his mind those arguments which support the view of his party, while it will infallibly prevent him from realising the force of the arguments propounded by the opposite side. Now it should be observed that the individual himself is probably quite unaware of this mechanism in his mind. He fondly imagines that his opinion is formed solely by the logical pros and cons of the measure before him. We see, in fact, that not only is his thinking determined by a complex of whose action he is unconscious, but he believes his thoughts to be the result of other causes which are in reality insufficient and illusory. This latter process of self-deception, in which the individual conceals the real foundation of his thought by a series of adventitious props, is termed 'rationalisation'.

The two mechanisms which manifest themselves in our example of the politician, the unconscious origin of beliefs and actions, and the subsequent process of rationalisation to which they are subjected, are of fundamental importance in psychology. They may be observed every day in every individual. That a man generally knows why he thinks in a certain way, and why he does certain things, is a widespread and cherished belief of the human race. It is, unfortunately, for the most part an erroneous one. We have an overwhelming need to believe that we are acting rationally, and are loath to admit that we think and do things without being ourselves aware of the motives producing those thoughts and actions. Now a very large number of our mental processes are the result of an emotional bias or complex of the type we have described. Such a causal chain is, however, incompatible with our ideal of rationality. Hence we tend to substitute for it a fictitious logical process, and persuade ourselves that the particular thought or action is its reasonable and natural result. This is the mechanism of rationalisation seen in the example of the politician; we shall meet with further illustrations of its effects throughout the whole sphere of normal and abnormal psychology.

The prevalence of 'rationalisation' is responsible for the erroneous belief that reason, taken in the sense of logical deduction from given premisses, plays the dominating role in the formation of human thought and conduct. In most cases the thought or action makes its appearance without any such antecedent process, moulded by the various complexes resulting from our instincts and experience. The 'reason' is evolved subsequently, to satisfy our craving for rationality.

The mechanism of rationalisation is most evident, perhaps, in the sphere of moral conduct, where we tend always to ascribe our actions to a conscious application of certain general religious or ethical principles. The majority of such actions are the result of habit, obedience to the traditions of our class, and other similar causes, and are carried out instinctively and immediately. The general principle is only produced subsequently, when we are challenged to explain our conduct. When the principle and the action do not entirely accord with each other, we amend the former by further rationalisations until it is capable of posing as the explanation of the latter, and in this way preserve our ideal of rationality. Thus it is a familiar fact that people of otherwise irreproachable honesty will swindle the government or a railway company with untroubled equanimity. If they are taxed with the incongruity between their principles and their conduct, a varied crop of rationalisations will be immediately produced. They will point out that a company is not the same thing as an individual, that nobody really loses anything, that the fares or taxes are so inequitable that it is justifiable to evade them, and so on. The distinction between the real and apparent causes of mental processes is well illustrated in the advice given to the newly created judge, 'Give your decision, it will probably be right. But do not give your reasons, they will almost certainly be wrong.'

It will be obvious, therefore, that to ask a man why he does a certain thing is by no means an invariably efficient method of discovering the genuine causes underlying his action. Introspection, however honestly it may be carried out, frequently fails when it attempts more than the mere recording of the superficial contents of consciousness. So soon as it aims at the elucidation of the real springs of action, there is always the possibility that either no result whatever is obtainable, or one vitiated by the mechanism of rationalisation. This fact is of primary importance, even to the psychologist who concerns himself only with the normal mind. For the investigator who extends his researches to the sphere of the abnormal, it possesses a significance which cannot be overestimated. That significance will be better appreciated, however, when we have proceeded further in our discussion of the action of complexes.

Various elaborate methods have been devised by which this difficulty in investigation may be overcome, and by which the complexes really responsible for the mental processes present may be laid bare. For the most part they require considerable knowledge and experience before they can be satisfactorily employed, and any adequate description of the procedure necessary is altogether impossible within the limits of this book. We may be permitted, however, to digress for a moment into the field of experimental psychology, and to devote a few words to the interesting method introduced by Jung, which is of great service in psychological investigations.

A list of words is read out to the patient, and in response to each he is required to give the first word which occurs to him. The word read out is known as the stimulus word, and the patient's reply is termed the reaction word. Generally it is found that the latter is related to the former by some simple associative link. Thus, to the stimulus word 'table' the reaction word 'chair' might be given, or some other simple association of a similar character. The time elapsing between the calling out of the stimulus word and the patient's reply is known as the reaction time, and is carefully measured by means of a stop-watch.

Now Jung found that the reaction obtained varied considerably, according as the stimulus word had or had not aroused a complex to activity. The reactions characteristic of the activity of a complex exhibited increase of the reaction time and various peculiarities in the reaction word. The following example, given by Jung and Peterson, illustrates some of the points in question:

Stimulus word	Reaction word	Reaction time (sec.)
1 Head	Hair	1·4
2 Green	Meadow	1·6
3 *Water*	*Deep*	5·0
4 Stick	Knife	1·6
5 Long	Table	1·2
6 *Ship*	*Sink*	3·4
7 Ask	Answer	1·6

Stimulus word		Reaction word	Reaction time (sec.)
8	Wool	Knit	1·6
9	Spiteful	Friendly	1·4
10	*Lake*	*Water*	4·0
11	Sick	Well	1·8
12	Ink	Black	1·2
13	*Swim*	*Can swim*	3·8

The patient from whom this series was obtained had, during a recent attack of depression, determined to commit suicide by drowning. This complex had manifested itself in the associations which are italicised. 3, 6, 10, and 13 are instances of increased reaction time; 13 shows also a peculiarity in the reaction word itself.

As a result of his researches, Jung maintained that by means of the association experiment it was possible to obtain information concerning the principal complexes in the mind of a given subject. This method has now been considerably developed and elaborated. It is of great service in the preliminary investigation of a case, and often furnishes valuable indications of the directions along which a subsequent detailed analysis may most profitably be conducted.[1]

We must now resume the thread of our original inquiry, and continue our discussion of the mode in which the action of complexes is manifested in the production of thoughts and actions.

In the examples of the photographer and the politician the complex expresses itself directly, that is to say, the photography-complex causes the man to think 'photographically', the political-complex causes him to think politically. But often the complex expresses itself indirectly by some manifestation which at first sight seems altogether different in nature. We may illustrate the meaning of this statement by the following example: one of my patients, a former Sunday-school teacher,

[1] The subsequent history of the association test has not fulfilled the expectation that it would be of great value in the psychological analysis of patients. It still provides an interesting sphere of experimental investigation, but is only occasionally used in practical medical treatment.

had become a convinced atheist. He insisted that he had reached this standpoint after a long and careful study of the literature of the subject, and, as a matter of fact, he really had acquired a remarkably wide knowledge of religious apologetics. He discoursed at length upon the evidence of Genesis, marshalling his arguments with considerable skill, and producing a coherent and well-reasoned case. Subsequent psychological analysis, however, revealed the real complex responsible for his atheism; the girl to whom he had been engaged had eloped with the most enthusiastic of his fellow Sunday-school teachers. We see that in this patient the causal complex, resentment against his successful rival, had expressed itself by a repudiation of the beliefs which had formerly constituted the principal bond between them. The arguments, the study, and the quotations were merely an elaborate rationalisation.

Here is another example of indirect expression of a complex, occurring in the same case. The patient had been for some time on bad terms with his father, to whom he was, nevertheless, very sincerely attached. The father's persistent refusal to entertain any proposals of reconciliation was a source of great distress to my patient. On one occasion the latter came to me in an unusually depressed frame of mind. He stated that on the morning in question he had seen two foreigners badly treated, and the occurrence has so revolted him that he had felt completely upset for the remainder of the day. I was sufficiently acquainted with the psychology of his case to realise that the alleged cause was quite insufficient to account for the mental state present, and I therefore proceeded to a more thorough investigation. Analysis soon revealed the real causal complex. The patient had that morning received a letter from his father containing the usual abuses and reproaches. The actual cause of the depression was the ill-treatment which he had himself experienced from his father, the troubles of the two foreigners merely serving the purpose of a rationalisation.

As a simpler and more familiar example of indirect expression of a complex we may cite a case mentioned by Jung. A man walking with a friend in the neighbourhood of a country village, suddenly expressed extreme irritation concerning the church bells, which happened to be pealing at the moment. He maintained that their tone was intrinsically unpleasant, their harmony ugly, and the total effect altogether disagreeable. The friend was astonished, for the bells in question were famous for their singular beauty. He endeavoured, therefore, to elucidate the real cause underlying his companion's attitude. Skilful questioning elicited the further remark that not only were the bells unpleasant but the clergyman of the church wrote extremely bad poetry. The causal complex was then apparent, for the man whose ears had been offended by the bells also wrote poetry, and in a recent criticism his work had been compared very unfavourably with that of the clergyman. The rivalry-complex thus engendered had expressed itself indirectly by an unjustifiable denunciation of the innocent church bells. The direct expression would, of course, have been abuse of the clergyman himself or of his works.

It will be observed that, without the subsequent analysis, the behaviour of the man would have appeared inexplicable, or at best ascribable to 'bad temper', 'irritability', or some other not very satisfying reason. Most cases where sudden passion over some trifle is witnessed may be explained along similar lines, and demonstrated to be the effect of some other and quite adequate cause. The apparently incomprehensible reaction is then seen to be the natural resultant of perfectly definite antecedents.

It will be profitable here to interrupt our investigations for a moment, in order to consider the position now reached, and the possible inferences which may be drawn to aid us in our attack upon the problems of mental disorder. We have found that the processes of the normal mind are in part the result of causes or 'complexes', of whose action the individual himself may be altogether unconscious. Secondly, the action of such complexes may be indirect, so that the conscious processes produced may have but little *prima facie* relation to the causes responsible for them. Thirdly, the individual may believe his thoughts or actions to be the results of other causes, which have in reality played no part whatever in their production, but are only the effects of a subsequent process of rationalisation.

These various mechanisms will obscure, both for himself and for the observer, the efficient causes responsible for the individual's train of thought or action. The efficient causes will not be those lying upon the surface, but deeper processes only to be unravelled by a delicate psychological analysis. Now it is possible that mechanisms of a similar nature may play a part in the production of the symptoms of insanity, and that these symptoms may be the indirect and distorted expressions of hidden complexes. In that case their apparent incomprehensibility would be due merely to our ignorance of these complexes and would vanish so soon as the latter were unearthed. The exaggerated misery of the melancholic patient over some inadequate and absurd idea would lose its appearance of inadequacy and absurdity if we could demonstrate that it was really the result of some other and quite efficient cause, just as the incomprehensible irritation, apparently produced in Jung's patient by the church bells, was fully explained when the underlying mental processes were laid bare. Similarly the delusions exhibited by some of our patients might not seem such grotesque and baseless anomalies if we ceased to take them at their face value, and insisted on delving deeper into the mind. Possibly we should then discover them to be merely indirect expressions, or perhaps attempts at rationalisation, of underlying processes which in themselves might be perfectly reasonable and coherent.

The hypothesis that the insane mind is not the chaos which a superficial observer imagines it to be, but that the appearance of disorder is due only to our ignorance of the deeper mental processes which link up the disjointed symptoms into a coherent whole, is at any rate suggestive and stimulating. Subsequent chapters will show, as a matter of fact, that recent psychological researches justify and confirm it to a very large extent. We shall hope to demonstrate that the thoughts and actions of the insane are not a meaningless and inscrutable medley, but that cause and effect play as considerable a part in the mind of the apparently incomprehensible insane patient as in that of the normal man. We shall find reason to believe, moreover, that not only are the mental processes of the insane explicable by psychological laws, but these laws are identical with those governing the minds of the sane, that the insane patient is battling with the same troubles which beset us all, and that he is endeavouring to express ideas, desires, and ambitions, with which we are all acquainted.

CHAPTER VI

CONFLICT

WE have described in the last chapter certain psychological laws which are constantly to be found in action both in the normal and in the insane mind. An attentive examination of the phenomena in which those laws are manifested, will convince us, however, that the position so far reached can in no sense be regarded as final. Further problems at once suggest themselves. Why is an individual sometimes aware of the complexes determining his thoughts and actions, and sometimes not so aware? Why does a complex in one instance express itself simply and immediately, in another by those devious routes which we have termed 'indirect'? Why does the father's letter make my patient miserable about the two foreigners, instead of making him miserable about the father's treatment of himself? The answers to these questions involve two further psychological conceptions, those of 'conflict' and 'repression'. These conceptions are of fundamental importance, and it will be necessary to examine them at considerable length.

Suppose that a complex is for some reason out of harmony with the mind as a whole, perhaps because of its intrinsically painful nature, perhaps because it prompts to actions which are incompatible with the individual's general views and principles. In such a case a state of 'conflict' arises, a struggle, as it were, between the complex and the personality.[1] These two forces will tend mutually to inhibit each other, the mind will be divided against itself, and a paralysis of action will

---

[1] 'Personality' is used here to denote all the mental processes—ideas, emotions, memories, desires—which do not belong to the complex in question. That is to say, it denotes the whole of the mind with the exception of the particular complex which is under discussion at the moment. This division of the mind into two parts is only a more exact description of that currently implied when, for example, we speak of a man conquering, or acceding to, a desire or temptation.

ensue. The conception of conflict may be illustrated by an adaptation of our former example of the lover. Let us assume that the object of his passion is already the wife of another man. The lover's mind will then exhibit two complexes trending in opposite and incompatible directions, on the one hand the desire for the woman, on the other the opposing tendencies constituted by moral education and fear of consequences. Under such circumstances neither is able to express itself freely in appropriate action, and a state of conflict results. This state of conflict is characterised by a condition of unpleasant emotional tension: the individual feels himself torn between two lines of conduct, neither of which is possible on account of the resistance offered by the other.

Conflict, with its emotional tension and accompanying indecision and paralysis of action, cannot persist indefinitely; it is a biological necessity that some solution of the difficulty, some way out of the *impasse*, should be found. This necessary solution may be attained in many different ways. For example, the complex may be modified so that its incompatibility with the personality no longer exists, or the mind may clearly recognise that the two possible ends cannot both be achieved and, after due weighing of the merits of each, consciously decide that one must be abandoned in favour of the other.

This subjective appreciation of the forces at war within us, and deliberate adoption of a consciously selected line of conduct, may be regarded as the rational or ideal solution of a conflict. In fact it may be said to provide the only possible solution in the strict sense of the word. In those other methods which we are now about to describe, the mind rids itself of the emotional tension and paralysis of action, not by a fight to a finish, but by a process of *avoiding* the conflict altogether. The mind is saved from the stress and strain of battle, because the two antagonists are not allowed to meet.

The first of these methods consists in the simple expedient of preserving both the opposing groups of ideas in the mind, while at the same time all contact or interaction between them is sedulously avoided. Each is allowed to pursue its own course and development, untroubled by its incongruity with the other. A mind exhibiting this phenomenon may be compared to an orchestra where one instrumentalist plays some independent melody of his own choosing, unconcerned by the discord he creates with the concerted harmony of his fellows. This is the common mechanism of the 'logic-tight compartment', which we have already met with in the chapter upon 'dissociation'. By its aid the man whose morality in private life is unimpeachable is enabled to practise a quite different moral code so far as his commercial transactions are concerned, because the two spheres of action are kept rigidly apart in his mind. It provides the explanation of the well-known antithesis between precept and practice, and enables us to understand that large section of the human race, often erroneously regarded as conscious hypocrites,

> Whose life laughs through and spits at their creed,
> Who maintain Thee in word, and defy Thee in deed.

The same mechanism explains the inability of the lover to appreciate the obvious imperfections of his lady: he cannot see them because his mind will not see them, the disturbing facts are not allowed to come into contact with his passions and the opinions which result therefrom. In a similar way we preserve the traditional beliefs of our childhood, whatever contradictory facts our experience may subsequently have presented to us. No conflict arises, because the beliefs and the facts live in separate logic-tight compartments of our minds, and are never permitted to come face to face in the field of consciousness.

It were easy to multiply indefinitely illustrations from normal life of this method of treating incompatible mental factors by the simple process of mutual exclusion. Honest introspection will no doubt furnish the reader with copious examples from his own mental life, or, if he finds this task insuperable, he will have no difficulty in observing the mechanism at work in the minds of his neighbours.

Here, however, we must pass on into the sphere of the abnormal, and endeavour to discover whether, and to what extent, this principle is evident in the phenomena of insanity. We find, as a matter of fact, that it plays a very large part in those phenomena, and that it renders intelligible a whole group of facts generally regarded as peculiarly characteristic of the insane. The patient who believes herself to be a queen, but who nevertheless cheerfully and contentedly carries out her daily task of scrubbing the ward, is not perturbed by the incongruity between her beliefs and conduct. The conflict between the two is avoided by the process of not allowing them to confront one another in the field of consciousness; the delusion is preserved in a logic-tight compartment secure from the disturbing influence of hard facts. By this means the complexes underlying the delusion, complexes whose nature we shall study at a subsequent stage of our investigations, succeed in obtaining expression in spite of the incompatible processes present in the remainder of the mind. Similarly those other cases mentioned at the conclusion of chapter IV—the patient who believes that he is the son of George III although he is at the same time perfectly aware of the actual past history of himself and his family, the patient who claims that he is omnipotent but who implores the gift of a little tobacco—these are all examples of the mechanism of the logic-tight compartment. In all of them contradictory systems of ideas are present in the mind, but conflict is avoided by allowing each system to develop independently, secure from contact with any idea or fact which may be incompatible therewith.

It will be remembered that in chapter IV these instances were cited as examples of dissociation. We have, therefore, now carried our investigation a stage further, and have discovered the mechanism upon which this dissociation depends. The mind has lost its homogeneity and is composed of more or less isolated mental processes, each pursuing its own independent course unaffected by the presence of its fellows, simply because those mental processes were contradictory and incompatible, and the conflict between them has been avoided by dissociating one from the others. The splitting of the mind has taken place because the two opponents could not be reconciled, and the device of permitting each to occupy its own logic-tight compartment afforded the easiest method of avoiding the otherwise inevitable conflict. From the standpoint now reached we may therefore lay down the principle that, in some cases at least, dissociation is the result of conflict, and that it is one of the methods by which the mind gets rid of the unpleasant emotional tension and paralysis of action that conflict invariably produces. The hypothesis immediately suggests itself, moreover, that all cases of dissociation, all those varying grades described in chapter IV, somnambulism, double personalities, obsessions, hallucinations, and delusions, may possibly be due to a similar mechanism. Dissociation would then always indicate the presence of a mental conflict, and would acquire the significance of a defensive reaction adopted by the mind when confronted with two incompatible systems of ideas. We shall subsequently find that a large number of varying grades of dissociation are, as a matter of fact, capable of being explained by this hypothesis, and that the evidence in its favour is very convincing. For the moment, however, it is necessary to retrace our steps and to modify in some degree certain of the principles already laid down.

It has been stated that a common method of avoiding conflict, in both the normal and the insane mind, consists in the process of dissociating the two opposing systems of ideas so that each is permitted to pursue its own development uninfluenced by its incongruity with the other. In the description of the examples used to illustrate this method it was further stated that a complex was thus segregated in a logic-tight compartment, into which no contradicting fact or idea was allowed to enter. That is to say, the complex preserves its freedom from conflict by simply neglecting altogether the significance of any fact or idea which is incompatible with it: contact between the two is completely avoided. Now although this statement is literally true of a small number of cases, the actual state of affairs is in most instances somewhat more complicated. Contact between the two opposing systems of ideas can rarely be avoided in the completely efficient manner which our description suggests. The opposing systems do come into contact, but only through a medium which so distorts the connecting processes that the real significance of the incompatible forces is concealed, and the mind fails to appreciate that any actual contradiction is present. This distorting medium is provided by the mechanism of rationalisation. Rationalisation, instances of which we have already met with in chapter IV, allows the mind to regard the facts incompatible with the complex in such a light that their incompatibility is more or less efficiently cloaked. This conception of two opposing groups of ideas, only allowed to come into contact through the distorting medium of rationalisation, will be made clearer by the consideration of some specific examples. The man whose commercial morality differs fundamentally from the code which he practises in his private life, persuades himself that the latter code is not properly applicable to business relations, that to ask a customer three times the value of a certain article is obviously something quite different from thieving, that a man must live, and that the immorality of lying completely disappears when it is necessary for the support of one's wife and family. Whenever, in fact, our actions conflict with our ethical principles we seek for specious reasons which will enable us to regard the actions in question as a peculiar case altogether justified by the circumstances in which they are carried out. The example cited in chapter v, of the honest man who swindles the railway company and the government without in any way injuring his sense of personal rectitude, provides an excellent illustration of the process we are now describing. In all these cases the incompatible systems of ideas are allowed to come into contact, but only by means of a bridge of rationalisations which so distorts their mutual significance that conflict is efficiently avoided. That is to say, the separate compartment of the mind in which the complex pursues its development is 'logic-tight', but not 'idea-tight'; opposing ideas are allowed to enter, but only after their logical significance has been distorted by a process of rationalisation.

If we now turn again to the sphere of the abnormal we shall

find that the mechanism of rationalisation plays a very prominent part. The patient who possesses a delusion neglects as far as possible the facts which are incompatible with his belief, but if he is compelled to take them into account he rationalises them in such a way that their actual significance is effectually concealed. Thus, the patient who is firmly convinced that his wife is seeking to murder him, will distort the meaning of everything which happens until it is brought into harmony with his dominating delusion, and capable of being used as a pseudo-logical prop. If his wife is solicitous for his welfare her behaviour is regarded as a cloak to conceal her real design, if she treats him badly the evil intentions are clear, if she gives him food it is obvious that she proposes to poison him, if she does not it is equally obvious that she hopes to undermine his health by withholding the necessaries of life. If we argue with him and point out that his belief is inconsistent with the facts, he smiles contemptuously at our credulity, or is perhaps suspicious that we are the paid accomplices of his wife.

This mechanism is responsible for a large group of the phenomena of insanity which may be termed 'secondary delusions'. 'Secondary delusions' are erroneous beliefs erected by the mind in order to bridge over the incongruity between the primary delusion and the actual facts of the patient's experience. For example, the patient who believes that he is a millionaire will meet the obvious fact that he has not a penny in his pocket by developing the further belief that he is the victim of an organised plot to deprive him of his property. Delusions of grandeur are, indeed, almost invariably accompanied by delusions of persecution. The patient cannot conceal from himself that his claims to exalted rank and position are not recognised by his environment, but he rationalises this failure of recognition by persuading himself that it is the work of a malignant and envious enemy. In this way the most complicated delusional systems may arise, the patient being convinced that more and more elaborate persecutions are being employed the more he meets with evidence contradicting the primary belief.

CHAPTER VII

REPRESSION

In the last chapter we have dealt with the general question of mental conflict, and have discussed one of the methods by which the mind may avoid the internal stress and accompanying disagreeable emotional tension which a state of conflict inevitably produces. This method, characterised by the formation in the mind of 'logic-tight compartments', accounts, as we have seen, not only for many of the phenomena observed in everyday life but also for some of the secondary phenomena met with in insanity.

Sometimes, however, this simple method of avoidance is not available, and the mind may then resort to other ways of freeing itself from the stresses and strains of conflict. The majority of these other methods are included under the general conception of 'repression', and we must now proceed to examine this conception and the various phenomena which it serves to explain.

The precise conditions under which the mechanism of the 'logic-tight compartment' can no longer be employed are at present imperfectly understood. The factors which play the principal part therein can, however, probably be summarised in the two following groups. First, the complexes at war with one another may be of such intrinsic importance and strength that the conflict between them cannot be concealed from the mind by the simple process of allowing each to pursue its own independent course and development. Secondly, the mind may be of a relatively more sensitive type which detects at once the unsatisfactory nature of this procedure. That is to say, the mind may be constitutionally endowed with a capacity for clear self-criticism, such that it is unable to delude itself by the easy mechanism of the logic-tight compartment, and cannot be satisfied by the very obvious rationalisations which that mechanism employs. Under these circumstances either the mind must face the conflict and fight it to a finish in the way we have previously described, or it must resort to the more elaborate methods of avoidance which are included under the conception of 'repression'.

In the method of the logic-tight compartment each of the opposing complexes is allowed a place in the field of consciousness. In the mechanism of repression, however, conflict is avoided by banishing one of the opponents from consciousness and no longer allowing it to achieve its normal expression, while the other opponent is left in possession of the field. This process of banishing a complex, so that it is prevented from appearing in consciousness, is the essential character of the mechanism of repression. Its nature will be best understood by the consideration of a simple example. Let us suppose that a man has in the past done some action of which he is now ashamed, so that every time the thought of this action recurs to him it occasions painful feelings of remorse. Expressing this state of affairs in our technical language, we should say that the memory of the action forms a complex which is repugnant to the personality as a whole, and that therefore a conflict is set up between the complex and the personality. Under such circumstances the individual may endeavour to rid himself of the feelings of remorse by striving to banish the painful memories from his mind, to keep them studiously out of his thoughts, and so far as possible to ignore their existence. That is to say, he may endeavour to avoid the conflict by 'repressing' the offending complex, and shutting it out from the field of consciousness. This method of attaining peace of mind by refusing to acknowledge to ourselves the existence of unpleasant facts which would otherwise grievously disquiet us will be familiar to everybody. Much of the 'forgetting' which occurs in our lives is not the passive process of decay which it is commonly supposed to be, but an active repression, a deliberate exclusion of the offending memory from the sphere of our consciousness.

In so far as the repression is successful the complex is

dislocated from the remainder of the mind, and thrown out of gear, as it were, with the personality. It is banished from the field of consciousness, and can no longer manifest itself there in the normal manner described in chapter v; that is to say, the complex can no longer cause the direct introduction into consciousness of the ideas, emotions, and trains of activity belonging to it.

Although the complex is thus forbidden to manifest itself in the field of consciousness, we assume, for reasons which will presently be clear, that it does not thereby cease to exist. The complex is not annihilated, but is shut out, and deprived of its normal functions. It persists in the deeper layers of the mind, as it were, although it is prevented from rising to the surface by the constant resistance which the repressive process opposes to it.

It will be evident that repression is/a more drastic method of dealing with conflict than that offered by the 'logic-tight compartment', and that its disturbing effect upon the homo-geneity and unity of the mind will be proportionally greater. Hence, although repression in its minor degrees is by no means uncommon in everyday life, for its more pronounced mani-festations we must turn to the sphere of the definitely abnor-mal. We shall, indeed, best achieve a clear understanding of its action by proceeding at once to those examples where repression produces its most marked effects. Such examples are provided by the cases described in chapter iii, under the headings of somnambulism and double personality.

Let us consider, in the light of the conceptions now at our disposal, the case of the patient Irène (p. 33). It will be remembered that Irène's mental troubles dated from the illness and death of her mother. The circumstances connected with the death were peculiarly painful, and the event pro-duced a profound shock upon Irène's mind. She had been deeply attached to her mother, and the latter had filled the chief place in all her thoughts, ambitions, and activities. Her mother's death, therefore, not only produced a great grief but deprived all those ambitions and activities of their main object and end. We may translate this state of affairs into our technical language as follows: the ideas connected with the mother's illness and death formed a system or complex intensely painful and repugnant to the personality as a whole. A conflict, with all its accompanying emotional stress and tension, was thus produced between the personality and the complex in question. To get rid of this conflict the mechanism of repression was brought into play. The painful complex was dislocated from the remainder of the mind, and no longer allowed to introduce its constituent ideas and emotions into the field of consciousness. Hence we find that Irène, in the intervals between her somnambulisms, had forgotten the whole system of ideas connected with her mother's death, and remembered nothing of the illness or its tragic end. She discussed her mother calmly, and as if nothing had happened to disturb the tenor of her own life. It will be seen, therefore, that the mechanism of repression had fulfilled its purpose: the conflict and its painful emotions were avoided, because one of the opposing complexes was altogether eliminated from the field of consciousness.

Now, it has been stated above that a complex which is thus repressed is not annihilated, but continues to exist in the deeper layers of the mind. The reasons which justify this hypothesis are clearly apparent in the case that we are now discussing. The complex which Irène has so efficiently repressed demonstrates its continued existence by suddenly erupting, as it were, and occupying for a time the whole field of consciousness. This is the state of affairs present during the periods of somnambulism. The system of ideas associated with the mother's illness suddenly makes its appearance and Irène lives once more through the whole tragic scene.

It must be carefully observed that, even during the somnambulisms, the mechanism of repression is still efficient. The complex which was formerly repressed is now in possession of the stage, but it possesses the whole stage, and all other ideas are temporarily abolished. While the somnambulism is in progress Irène is wholly absorbed in her phantasy, and altogether oblivious of her actual environment, and of what is taking place around her. That is to say, the complete dissociation between the opposing complexes which constitutes the essential feature of repression is still present, and the resistance which keeps them apart is as potent as ever. The complex which was formerly submerged is now able to express itself freely, but only because its opponent, represented here by the remainder of the personality, has in turn been shut out from the field of consciousness.

The conception of repression, therefore, enables us to explain yet another group of the dissociations of consciousness described in chapter IV. In the case of somnambulisms the complex underlying the dissociated system is in a state of repression, and deprived of its normal interplay with the remainder of the mind. It is, therefore, only able to express itself in the field of consciousness by the production of ideas and images which are sharply cut off from the remainder of the conscious stream. In other words, the ideas due to the activity of the complex form a completely segregated or dissociated group.

It has been pointed out, in chapter IV, that the condition known as 'double personality' differs from somnambulism only in degree. In both cases we are dealing with systems of ideas which are completely dissociated from the remainder of the mind, but in double personality the dissociated system is more complicated and complete in its structure, so that while it occupies the stage, the individual is still able to adapt himself to his environment, and does not exhibit that absolute oblivion of the real world which characterises the somnambulist.

In view of this similarity, we may assume that the explanation given for somnambulisms is probably also applicable to double personalities, and that these dissociations are likewise due to a conflict between incompatible complexes which has been solved by a process of repression. As a matter of fact, such an explanation has been successfully applied to a considerable number of cases. Limitations of space, however, do not permit of any satisfactory description of them here.

It has been stated above that the group of dissociations, comprising somnambulisms and other closely allied phenomena, shows us the mechanism of repression in its clearest and most pronounced form. Repression, however, manifests itself in many other ways which, though less obvious and drastic than the methods just described, will be more familiar to the student of everyday life. These other manifestations form the subject-matter of the following chapter.

CHAPTER VIII

MANIFESTATIONS OF REPRESSED COMPLEXES

IN the last chapter it has been explained that when a complex is repressed it is thereby deprived of its normal mode of expression. That is to say, it can no longer cause its constituent ideas and emotions to enter directly into consciousness, and it can no longer cause the conscious stream to move along a course which will satisfy its own ends. These effects are produced because a certain resistance, or 'censure' as it is technically termed, is opposed to the normal action of the complex. Our understanding of this conception will perhaps be assisted

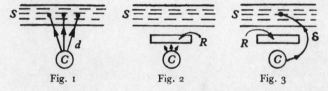

Fig. 1   Fig. 2   Fig. 3

by the consideration of the above diagrams which must, of course, be regarded as purely schematic.

Fig. 1 represents the normal action of a complex. S is the stream of consciousness, the succession of thoughts, emotions, and volitions which occupy the surface, as it were, of our minds. S corresponds, in fact, to the mind as it appears to ordinary introspection. C is a complex, and d represents the various ideas, etc., which the complex throws into the stream of consciousness so soon as it is stimulated in the manner described in chapter v.

Fig. 2 represents the state of affairs which arises if the complex is subjected to repression. A resistance (R) is now opposed to the normal action of the complex, so that the ideas belonging to the latter can no longer be thrown directly into the conscious stream in the manner shown in Fig. 1. Fig. 2 will, for example, illustrate the conditions present in Irène's mind during the interval between her somnambulisms. In this case C would represent the complex connected with the mother's illness and death. Owing to the presence of the resistance (R), all the ideas belonging to that complex would be absolutely cut off from the stream of consciousness, and we should have that localised loss of memory which Irène actually exhibited during the periods in question.

It was further stated in the preceding chapter that, although the repressed complex is thus deprived of its normal mode of expression, it does not thereby cease to exist. We must now add that it not only continues to exist, but continues to find expression, although that expression is no longer normal and direct. In the case of Irène the complex achieved expression by so interrupting the stream of consciousness that the portion of the stream in which it appeared, i.e. the somnambulism, was absolutely cut off from that which preceded it and from that which followed it. More generally, however, the mode of expression is less drastic than this, and is of the type shown in Fig. 3. The repressed complex cannot affect consciousness in the normal direct manner, but it nevertheless contrives to exert an influence along the devious and indirect path represented by δ. This path must be sufficiently devious and indirect to enable the complex to elude, as it were, the resistance (R), and the stronger the resistance the more indirect must the path of expression become.

The actual facts corresponding to the scheme shown in Fig. 3 will be rendered clear by the consideration of a specific instance, and for this purpose we may select the example borrowed from Dr Jung which was described upon p. 61. A certain man expressed extreme annoyance at some irreproachable church bells. Investigation revealed the fact that the man and the clergyman who was attached to the church were rivals in the field of amateur poetry. Now the causal complex responsible for the phenomena evidently originated in jealousy of a successful rival. But jealousy of this kind is an emotion whose existence we are rarely ready to acknowledge, even to ourselves. In other words, it forms a complex which is almost invariably repressed so far as we are able. A resistance is imposed which prevents the complex making its appearance in the field of consciousness. Hence the complex is compelled to express itself by some indirect path which will enable it to elude the resistance. In the present case this indirect path was provided by an unjustified criticism of the bells which were closely connected with the offending clergyman. By this means the complex found expression, while the individual was able to persuade himself that his action was due to a quite different cause. The resistance served its purpose by protecting consciousness from the direct manifestation of the unacknowledged complex, so that the conflict which would otherwise have arisen was avoided.

A similar explanation may be applied to the case, described on p. 61, of the patient who was so distressed at the ill-treatment meted out to two foreigners. The causal complex was the resentment which the patient felt at the ill-treatment that he had himself received from his father. But this complex was repressed because it was incompatible with the deep affection which he entertained for his father, and because a distressing conflict would otherwise have inevitably been engendered. Hence it obtained expression in the indirect manner described, by attaching its constituent emotion to an external event connected with the real cause by a relation of superficial similarity. The other examples of indirect expression of a complex cited in chapter IV are explicable along similar lines.

At the beginning of chapter VI the problem presented itself as to why a complex should in one case express itself simply and directly, in another by the devious routes termed 'indirect'. This problem we are now in a position to answer. A complex will express itself directly when it is not subjected to repression. A repressed complex, on the other hand, can influence the stream of consciousness only along an indirect path, because of the resistance which is offered by the 'censure'. Owing to this resistance the manifestations must be so distorted that its real origin in the tabooed complex is no longer apparent to the individual. Hence, whenever indirect expression of a complex is observed, it may be assumed that incompatible and conflicting systems of ideas are present in the mind, and that the complex in question is subjected to some degree of repression.

Now the solution of a mental conflict by the mechanism of repression is one of the commonest refuges of the human mind. We shall find that it not only explains the occurrence of phenomena frequently seen in everyday life, but also enables us to understand the genesis of many abnormal mental symptoms which are observed in the sphere of insanity. It will therefore be necessary to consider this mechanism in considerable detail.

A study of the diagrams on p. 78 will suggest to us that the phenomena caused by the presence of a repressed complex will be of two kinds. Either they will be indirect expressions of the complex itself, or they will be phenomena due to the resistance or 'censure' which forbids the complex to obtain its normal and direct expression. As a matter of fact we shall find that most of the symptoms produced by the mechanism of repression are clearly referable to one or other of these varieties. A simple example will render intelligible both the nature of the phenomena we are now considering, and the subdivision which we are seeking to establish. In certain elderly unmarried women the 'sex complex' (including in that term the various instincts belonging to sex) has been denied its normal outlet and has ultimately become repressed. Under these circumstances the existence of the repressed complex may be evidenced by two groups of familiar phenomena. The resistance which forbids the normal expression of the complex may appear as an exaggerated prudery; this clearly serves to conceal the objectionable complex from consciousness, and hence fulfils the function of a censure. The complex will contrive, nevertheless, to express itself in some indirect manner, e.g. as a morbid interest in births, marriages, and scandals.

Phenomena due to indirect expression and those ascribable to the censure will, of course, generally occur together, although in one case the first may be more prominent, in another the second. For purposes of description, however, it will be clearer to deal with the two groups separately, and we shall find it advantageous to commence with the consideration of the second group.

The essential character of the symptoms ascribable to the censure is that they assist the process of resistance, and help in the active repression of the objectionable complex. Availing ourselves of the diagrams on p. 78, we may regard these symptoms as weights added to the repressing process represented by R, which further guard against any appearance of the complex in the field of consciousness. In a large number of cases they are of the type seen in the prudery example described above, the exaggerated appearance in the superficial layers of the mind of the opposite quality to that belonging to the complex in question. A familiar instance is the concealment of diffidence and social shyness by the assumption of a boisterous good fellowship. In the sphere of insanity a similar mechanism accounts for some of the manic states described in chapter III. In a case recorded by Dr Devine, for example, the patient was suffering from an incurable cancer. She was at first intensely depressed, tortured by the pain accompanying the disease, and filled with gloomy forebodings concerning the future of her husband and children. Later, however, signs of excitement appeared, and finally she passed into a typical manic state, which necessitated her removal to the mental hospital. She was then abnormally joyous and elated, in constant movement, singing hymns and litanies, and apparently ecstatically happy. She maintained that she was now perfectly well, and that the disease had been completely cured. The psychological explanation of this case is obvious. The distressing conflict between the hopeless facts and all the patient's most cherished ambitions and desires, actually seen in the first phase of the case, had been solved by a process of repression. The facts were shut out from consciousness, and the resistance to their entry assisted by the development in consciousness of the abnormal gaiety and elation which characterised the manic phase. A similar mechanism probably accounts for the condition known as *spes phthisica*, the astonishing cheerfulness and optimism which frequently characterises the last stages of pulmonary consumption.

Another familiar manifestation of the censure is to be found in the concealment of a gnawing sorrow by the assumption of a witty exterior. It is a common observation that a secret unhappiness often lurks beneath the sparkling witticisms of the man of jokes. Humour is, indeed, one of the great refuges of life, and the man who is sensitive but has no humour suffers much from the bitterness of experience. By the aid of humour, experience which is unpalatable can be deprived of its real significance and treated as a joke, and thus we may be saved the sting of many a painful conflict. The extension of this principle into the field of abnormal psychology is perhaps best seen in the 'drunkard's humour', which is so characteristic a feature of the chronic alcoholic. Here we find a superficial wit, consisting essentially in an inability to take anything seriously, even the gravest facts of life. The consequences of his vice, poverty, a wrecked career, the miseries of wife and children, are glossed over by the alcoholic with a pleasantry or a *bon mot*, and are not allowed to disturb his exaggerated self-complacency. In this manner he achieves a superficial peace of mind, and is saved from that remorse which constitutes the most distressing of all conflicts.

The repression of a painful complex by the exaggerated development in consciousness of the opposite quality will also enable us to understand the genesis of some obsessions. The following example will serve as a minor illustration of this process. A man who had been addicted in his boyhood to the thieving of small sums of money, developed in later life an exaggerated honesty. He would devote endless time and trouble to the payment of some trifling excess fare, and an undischarged debt was a source of unceasing worry and self-reproach. The explanation of this abnormal rectitude is evidently to be found in the mechanism we are now considering. The memory of his early lapses constituted a painful complex intensely repugnant to the man's adult consciousness. He therefore strove to banish it from his mind, and to conceal its presence by the exaggerated assumption of the opposing quality. It will be remembered that in chapter III this over-weighting of a particular element in consciousness was described as the essential character which defines an obsession. Such obsessions may in some cases be so persistent and pronounced as altogether to upset the mental stability of the individual, so that his behaviour becomes definitely abnormal. A common example is 'washing mania', an irresistible desire to wash the hands at every moment of the day, with an over-whelming fear of dirt and contamination. This is often found where some morally objectionable habit is present which arouses constant remorse in the mind of the patient. The personality reacts to the complex, which it regards as morally unclean, by the symbolical assumption of an over-conscientious and exaggerated cleanliness.

In the majority of the examples hitherto considered the censure has manifested itself by the exaggerated development in consciousness of a quality which is the reverse of that present in the offending complex. It is not necessary, however, that the quality developed should always have this opposite character. Provided that it serves to conceal the complex it will efficiently carry out the repressing function for which it has been created. Cynicism, for instance, by which the individual endeavours to persuade himself that the complex or the forces which oppose it are worthless and unreal, is a common method of dealing with the insoluble conflicts of life. The artificial elation produced by alcohol, opium, and some other drugs, serves a similar purpose. The submerging of conflicts is, indeed, the chief object for which these drugs are taken, and this basic fact must be taken into account in any efficient attempt to deal with the alcohol question. It has been well said that

almost universally regarded as either, on the one hand, a sin or a vice, or, on the other hand, as a disease, there can be little doubt that it [alcoholism] is essentially a response to a psychological necessity. In the tragic conflict between what he has been taught to desire and what he is allowed to get, man has found in alcohol, as he has found in certain other drugs, a sinister but effective peacemaker, a means of securing, for however short a time, some way out of the prison-house of reality back to the Golden Age.[1]

Another way in which the resistance offered by consciousness to an offending complex may manifest itself, is by the assumption of some feverish activity, whose object is so to fill the field of consciousness with other ideas and activities that the repressed complex cannot make any appearance. A case in point is provided by the disappointed man who devotes himself to some strenuous sport or profession in order, as common language aptly expresses it, 'to drive his troubles from his mind'. A minor example of the same mechanism is often seen in everyday social life, when some subject peculiarly painful to one of the individuals present is inadvertently introduced into a general conversation. The individual may endeavour to conceal his perturbation by a rapid flow of remarks about some other thing, a phenomenon which may be described as a 'press of conversation'. A precisely similar mode of reaction, though more advanced in degree, accounts for certain symptoms met with in the sphere of insanity. Thus the symptom known as *vorbeireden*, a term which has been somewhat clumsily rendered into English as 'talking past the point', is frequently encountered in cases where the patient possesses some complex which he is endeavouring to repress. The patient does not answer our questions but replies with some totally irrelevant remarks, which are often grotesquely inappropriate, and give to his conversation a characteristic aspect of meaningless incoherence. Thus one patient, in whose life a lady of the name of Green had played a very prominent part, replied to the question 'Do you know a Miss Green?' with, 'Green, that's green, that's blue, would you say that water is blue?' Occasionally the patient dissects the question into its constituent words or syllables, furnishing a string of irrelevant associations to each, and thereby avoiding any direct answer to

[1] W. Trotter, *Instincts of the Herd in Peace and War* (London, 1916).

the question as a whole. Often it can be shown that a patient converses normally except when a question which stimulates the hidden complex is given; his replies then exhibit the peculiar incoherence just described. The explanation of this mode of reaction is, of course, that the repression is thereby preserved, and the stimulation is not allowed to exert its normal effect, the appearance in consciousness of the ideas belonging to the complex.

The symptom known as 'mutism', although apparently directly opposite in character to the rapid flow of talk described above, often serves a precisely similar purpose. The patient preserves a rigid silence, and our questions meet with no response whatever. Occasionally this phenomenon is generalised, as it were, so that for months at a time no word passes the patient's lips.

We must now turn to the other group of phenomena caused by the presence of a repressed complex, those due to the indirect expression of the complex itself. Numerous examples have already been given in the earlier part of the present chapter. We may now pass on, however, to consider instances which exhibit this mechanism in a more pronounced form, and where the manifestations produced are more definitely abnormal.

Certain compulsive actions belonging to the group of obsessions may be mentioned here, of which an excellent example is furnished by the case described on p. 36. It will be remembered that the patient in question suffered from an irresistible compulsion to examine the number of every bank-note which came into her hands. Now the genesis of this compulsion will be apparent so soon as we are acquainted with details of the patient's history which were revealed by a psychological analysis. Some time previously the lady had fallen in love with a certain man whom she had met in a country hotel. One day she asked him to change a coin for her. The man complied with her wish and, putting the coin in his pocket, remarked that he would not part with it. This episode aroused hopes in the lady's mind that her affections were reciprocated, and she longed to know whether he would keep his word. Any money which came into her hands always recalled the scene in the hotel, and the emotions and desires with which it was associated. The man finally departed, however, without making any further advances, and ultimately the lady realised that the hopes she had entertained could have no fruition. The conflict which thus arose was dealt with by a process of repression. The lady strove to banish the painful chapter from her life and to forget that the desires associated with it had ever existed. The repression was successful, and the complex was not permitted to make any appearance in consciousness by way of the normal channels. The intense interest in money which passed through her hands persisted, however, affording a route by which the complex could obtain an indirect expression, and this indirect expression crystallised into that exaggerated preoccupation with the bank-note numbers, which formed the dominant symptom of the case.

In all the instances of indirect expression which have hitherto been considered it will be apparent that the essential feature of the process consists in the complex expressing itself along so devious a route that it is enabled to avoid the resistance offered by the censure. The mode of expression must be sufficiently indirect to ensure that the real origin of the ideas appearing in consciousness is efficiently concealed from the individual himself. That is to say, the repressed complex can only exert an influence upon consciousness provided that the influence is distorted to a greater or less degree.

The various methods by which this necessary distortion may be attained are exceedingly numerous, and have but little in common beyond the one fundamental factor that they serve to conceal from consciousness the real origin of the ideas appearing in it. We have already become acquainted with many of these methods, and the detailing of other varieties will form the subject of the remainder of this chapter, and of the whole of the next. The mechanism of indirect expression has, indeed, an importance which cannot be over-estimated. There can be little doubt that a vast number of the symptoms of

D *

insanity are explicable as instances of its action, and that in it is to be found the solution of the apparently incomprehensible and senseless character which attaches to many of those symptoms. The meaning of this general statement will become clearer at a later stage of our investigation, and it will be profitable to postpone its more detailed consideration until we have accumulated some further material.

One of the most important methods by which the distortion necessary for the expression of a repressed complex is obtained consists in the employment of symbolism. For example, in elderly unmarried women the repressed maternal instincts may find a distorted outlet in an exaggerated affection for dogs and cats. The function of the symbolisation is obviously the concealing of the real causal ideas from the consciousness of the individual. In everyday life feelings of self-importance, whose overt expression is forbidden by the traditions of social conduct, frequently manifest themselves by the employment of symbolisms. We may cite such examples as affectations of gait or dress, a pedantic phraseology, the adoption of a conversation as polysyllabic as possible, and of a handwriting decorated with innumerable flourishes. In insanity symbolism plays a prominent part. The instances we have just considered appear in an exaggerated form as the stilted phraseology replete with neologisms, and other ludicrous affectations and mannerisms so frequently met with in the adolescent insane.

The mechanism of symbolisation accounts for many of the curious phenomena known as 'stereotyped actions', of which several examples were given in chapter III. We may select one borrowed from Dr Jung. An old female patient, who had been an inmate of the hospital for many years, spent her whole existence in the performance of a single stereotyped action. She had never been heard to speak, and she never exhibited the faintest interest in anything that went on around her. All day long she sat in a huddled position, continuously moving her arms and hands in a manner resembling the action of a shoemaker who is engaged in sewing boots. During her waking hours this movement absorbed her whole attention, and it was carried out with unfailing regularity and monotony from one year's end to another. When her history was investigated it was found that as a young girl she had been engaged to be married, and that the engagement had been suddenly broken off. This event occasioned a great emotional shock, and she rapidly passed into the insane state which persisted throughout the remainder of her life. It was further elicited that the faithless lover had been a shoemaker by trade.

Armed with these facts we can easily reconstruct the psychological processes responsible for the symptoms which the patient exhibited. The sudden termination of the engagement caused a distressing conflict, which was finally solved by a process of repression. The affections and desires which had played so important a part in the patient's mind were repressed on account of their incompatibility with the world of fact, and were only allowed to appear in an indirect and distorted form. This indirect expression was provided by the stereotyped action which symbolised for the patient the whole system of ideas and emotions connected with her lost lover. The entire detachment from the real world, the failure to react in any way to her environment, and the other symptoms present in this case will be better understood at a later stage of our inquiry, and will be fully dealt with in a subsequent chapter (p. 115).

A frequent method by which a repressed complex obtains an indirect expression is afforded by the mechanism known as 'projection'. This method is so important, and appears in such protean forms, that it will be necessary to study it in some detail, and the whole of the next chapter will therefore be devoted to its consideration.

CHAPTER IX

PROJECTION

IN the preceding chapter the phenomena produced by the repression of a complex were divided into two groups, those due to the indirect expression of the complex itself, and those due to the presence of a resistance or censure which prevents the complex exercising its normal direct effect. In all the examples hitherto considered the symptoms present could without much difficulty be assigned to one or other of these two groups. It will nevertheless be obvious that this distinction is largely artificial, and that in the formation of each symptom the factors of indirect expression and resistance both take part. The symptoms may be regarded, in fact, as a compromise between the two factors in question. The complex struggles to express itself, while the resistance endeavours to prevent it achieving its end. The symptom is finally evolved as a compromise between the two opposing forces. In each of the examples cited in the last chapter, however, one of the two components seemed to play a preponderating part in the compromise produced, so that the symptom could be classified as belonging to the corresponding group.

The group of symptoms to which we must now direct our attention, those due to the mechanism of 'projection', exhibit this preponderance of one component to a less marked degree, and the phenomena belonging to it are best regarded as instances of compromise formation in which the parts played by the two opposing forces are approximately equal.

'Projection' may be defined as a peculiar reaction of the mind to the presence of a repressed complex, in which the complex or its effect is regarded by the personality as belonging no longer to itself, but as the production of some other real or imaginary individual. The meaning of this definition will be made clear by the consideration of some simple examples

People who possess some fault or deficiency of which they are ashamed are notoriously intolerant of that same fault or deficiency in others. Thus the parvenu who is secretly conscious of his own social deficiencies talks much of the 'bounders' and 'outsiders' whom he observes around him, while the one thing which the muddle-headed man cannot tolerate is a lack of clear thinking in other people. In general it may be said that whenever one encounters an intense prejudice one may with some probability suspect that the individual himself exhibits the fault in question or some closely similar fault. An excellent illustration of this mechanism is to be found in *Hamlet*, in the excessive aversion with which the Player-Queen regards the possibility of a second marriage, although a secret desire for such a marriage is already present in her mind.

> The instances that second marriage move
> Are base respects of thrift, but none of love . . .
> Nor earth to me give food, nor heaven light.
> Sport and repose lock from me day and night,
> To desperation turn my trust and hope,
> An anchor's cheer in prison be my scope,
> Each opposite that blanks the face of joy
> Meet what I would have well, and it destroy,
> Both here and hence pursue me lasting strife,
> If, once a widow, ever I be wife.

Shakespeare's acquaintance with the psychological mechanism we are considering is evidenced by the comment of the real queen:

> The lady doth protest too much, methinks.

We may express the psychological processes seen in these cases as follows; the fault constitutes a complex which is repugnant to the personality as a whole, and its presence would therefore naturally lead to that particular form of conflict which is known as self-reproach. The personality avoids this conflict, however, by 'projecting' the offending complex on to some other person, where it can be efficiently rebuked without that painful emotion which inevitably accompanies the recognition of deficiencies in ourselves. That is to say, the personality reacts to the repugnant complex by exaggeratedly reproaching the same facts in other people, thereby concealing the skeleton in its own cupboard. The more comfortable expedient of rebuking one's neighbour is substituted for the unpleasant experience of self-reproach. The biological function served by projection is, therefore, the same as in all other varieties of repression, the avoidance of conflict and the attainment of a superficial peace of mind.

In the sphere of insanity the mechanism of projection plays a prominent part, and a great variety of symptoms may be ascribed to its action. Alcoholism, described in the last chapter as one of humanity's refuges from the stress of conflict, provides many excellent examples. The chronic alcoholic develops with great frequency delusions concerning the conduct of his wife or other relatives. Thus one of my patients complained bitterly that his wife was dissolute, a drunkard, and a spendthrift, that she neglected both himself and the children, and that she allowed the home to go to rack and ruin. Investigation showed, however, that all these ideas were purely delusional, and without foundation in fact. The patient himself was the real culprit, and each statement that he made was true of himself but not of his wife. The psychological explanation of his delusions is to be found in the mechanism of projection. By its aid the patient's personality was enabled to treat the objectionable complex as an entire stranger for whom it was in no sense responsible, and thereby to substitute an illusory self-complacency for the pangs of remorse. In such cases as these alcoholism has indeed achieved its aim, and freedom from conflict has been attained, but only at the price of mental integrity and self-honesty, and the mental hospital has become the inevitable consequence.

Many so-called 'delusions of persecution' may be similarly explained by the mechanism of projection. The patient has some secret desire which is repugnant to the personality, perhaps because it is incompatible with the individual's general principles or trends of thought. The mind, therefore refuses to treat the desire as part of itself, and projects it into some other real or fictitious person, who then becomes an enemy striving to achieve the patient's downfall. In its minor degrees this mechanism is to be seen in the excuses with which we frequently endeavour to mitigate our moral lapses. We will not acknowledge to ourselves that it was our own ambitions and desires which led to the commission of the fault, but seek to shift the blame to the shoulders of our neighbour. Through all ages 'the woman tempted me' has been a stock excuse of erring man. This type of projection attains a much greater development, however, in certain varieties of insanity. In 'old maids' insanity', for example, an unmarried lady of considerable age, and of blameless reputation, begins to complain of the undesirable attentions to which she is subjected by some male acquaintance. She explains that the man is obviously anxious to marry her, and persistently follows her about. Finally, certain trifling incidents lead her to believe that he is scheming to abduct her by force, and on the strength of this she perhaps writes him an indignant letter, or lodges a complaint with the police. Investigation follows, and it is found not only that the man is entirely innocent of the charges levelled against him, but that he has never expressed the least interest in the lady, and is probably hardly aware of her existence. The lady is certified to be suffering from 'delusions of persecution', and is removed to a hospital.

This by no means uncommon sequence of events can be easily explained with the aid of the psychological laws now at our disposal. The patient's sex instincts have been allowed no normal outlet, and have finally become sternly repressed, generally with an exaggerated development in consciousness of the opposite quality. This latter, of course, constitutes the prudery so frequently observed in such cases, whose origin we have studied in a former chapter. The repressed instincts obtain an indirect expression, however, by the mechanism of projection. The desires originating therefrom are roused to activity by the man in question, and the real state of affairs is that the lady is in love with the man but, owing to the repression, the mind will not acknowledge that these ideas and emotions are part of itself, and finds a solution of the conflict by reversing the significance of the desires and projecting them upon their own object. The bearer of the repugnant complex hence appears to the personality as an unwelcome aggressor, and the genesis of the persecutory delusions is complete.

In many cases of delusions of persecution in which the development is closely similar to that just described, the desires are projected into an individual who has no real existence. The patient's mind, in its struggle to obtain freedom from the internal conflict, invents not only the man's conduct, but the man himself. This more complicated form of projection is of common occurrence, and the female patient who indignantly complains of the violent wooing to which she is subjected by some altogether imaginary man is to be found in every mental hospital.

In another variety of projection it is not the complex itself which is projected but the reproaches to which it gives rise. The biological purpose which this variety subserves is the same as before, the avoidance of conflict. It is obvious that the painful stress which accompanies self-reproach is obviated so long as the two opposing forces whose conflict produces it are dislocated from each other, and this dislocation may be equally well attained by projecting either of the two antagonists. In the variety we are now about to consider the patient no longer reproaches himself, but imagines that he is being reproached by other people. The normal analogue of this process is well known—the guilty conscience which sees the accusing finger everywhere around. It is but a small step further to the development of 'delusions of reference'. The patient is intensely suspicious; if two or three of his fellows converse together he imagines that he forms the subject of the remarks, the casual stranger becomes a designing enemy, until finally every trivial event is welded into one vast conspiracy to destroy him. In patients of this kind the development of hallucinations is extremely common. The reproaches are not merely construed into the actions of those about them, they are handed over to altogether imaginary persecutors. The portion of his mind which the personality has cut off and declined to acknowledge makes its reappearance as an hallucinatory voice. Thus one patient, whose mode of life had wrecked both himself and his family, discussed his former experiences with revolting complacency. He complained bitterly, however, of the system of persecution to which he was subjected; people concealed themselves in the ceiling and under his bed, and poured upon him a flood of abuse and threats, which rendered existence almost insupportable. Hallucinations of this kind may be regarded as literal examples of the 'small voice of conscience', distorted by repression. It will be observed that such a patient has successfully avoided the sting of remorse, but he has exchanged Scylla for Charybdis, and has sacrificed his mental integrity to obtain the hardly more desirable alternative of a constant persecution.

In chapter IV it was pointed out that hallucinations, and the systems of ideas which hallucinations express, are to be regarded as dissociated portions of the patient's own consciousness. We are now in a position to understand why this dissociation takes place. The systems of ideas in question are for one reason or another incompatible with the personality as a whole, and their appearance in consciousness would in the ordinary course of events give rise to conflict and painful stress. To avoid this conflict repression has been called into play, and the repressed complexes can only obtain the indirect expression afforded by projection. The phenomena due to the projection are hence dislocated from the personality, and make their appearance as dissociated systems.

CHAPTER X

THE IRRATIONALITY OF THE INSANE

THE attribute of the insane patient which is at once the most general, the most obvious, and the most striking, is his apparent irrationality. It is so evident that the delusions he exhibits are false beliefs, that the hallucinations have no objective reality, that the depression or exaltation is totally unjustified by the actual state of affairs. He is, moreover, so plainly impervious to the contradictions which his experience everywhere presents to him, and so absurdly obtuse to every argument and demonstration which our wits can devise. In the face of all this the superficial observer can only conclude that the root of the evil lies in the patient's incapacity to see reason, and that these grotesque symptoms have arisen simply because the mind has lost its ability to think rationally. To such an observer the essence of the matter is that the reasoning powers are diseased, and hence that the mind is capable of thinking any thought, however absurd and baseless it may be.

A more careful investigation, however, soon reveals facts which it is difficult to reconcile with this view. In many patients the reasoning powers seem to be in excellent order so long as they are applied to matters not immediately connected with the delusional system. Thus a patient who is firmly convinced that he is the son of George III may be capable of solving the most abstruse mathematical problems, and may perhaps fulfil duties in the hospital which demand the utmost nicety of judgment and discrimination. Are we to assume that in such a case the reasoning powers act normally and efficiently so long as the question of the patient's ancestry is not touched upon, but that they then suddenly become diseased and useless, so that the mind is permitted to weave ludicrous ideas without being called to account at the bar of reason? Or are we to conclude that the theory of the superficial observer is not applicable, and that the fault does *not* lie in a disease of the reasoning powers?

A consideration of the results reached in the preceding chapters of this book enables us at once to decide in favour of the second alternative. The origin of the abnormal mental processes is not to be found in any disturbance of the reasoning powers *per se*, but in the material which is presented to those powers. The patient does not believe that he is the son of George III because he has lost the capacity to reason, but because the proposition is presented to his mind in a light which makes it the only plausible and rational conclusion possible. He is only apparently irrational, because the observer does not see the chain of mental processes which have produced the result, but only the result itself, standing as an isolated phenomenon without obvious basis or justification.

The apparent absurdity of the delusion rests on the fact that it is the indirect expression of some other mental process which is itself hidden from view. This other process is intelligible and understandable enough, once it has been elicited. So long as it remains hidden, however, the delusion must inevitably appear to be a structure without foundation, and without relation to things as they are. The analyses contained in preceding chapters will all serve to illustrate the truth of this proposition. We found that in every case the incomprehensibility of the delusion disappeared so soon as we unearthed the chain of mental processes actually responsible for it, just as the man who falls into a passion over some trifle is incomprehensible only until we discover that his rage is really the result of some other and quite adequate cause.

We can understand, moreover, the well-known fact that it is useless to argue with the insane patient concerning his delusions. As our arguments will be directed, not against the hidden real cause of the delusion; but merely against its superficial manifestation, they will obviously be ineffective. Their only result will be to stimulate the patient to produce 'rationalisations', endeavours to establish illusory logical props for a structure which is really built upon the underlying complex.

This method of dealing with arguments is not peculiar to the insane. Examples of its employment are to be seen everywhere around us, and it has become proverbial in the couplet—

> A man convinced against his will
> Is of the same opinion still.

Translated into technical language this would read: 'It may be possible by argument to show that each rationalisation which the man produces is logically untenable, until finally he can produce no more—but as the complex really responsible for his position has not been attacked at all, it continues to produce its effect, and the man remains of the same opinion.' The futility of logic as a weapon against the products of a complex is notorious. No one imagines that it is possible to alter the convictions of a zealous party politician or sectarian by the process of arguing with him. For precisely the same reasons no psychiatrist imagines that argument is of any avail against the delusions of the insane. In both cases the individual becomes credulous or blind, according as the arguments produced agree or conflict with the trend of the underlying complex.

If we are called upon to explain the imperviousness to argument of the enthusiastic party politician or sectarian, we do not assume that it is dependent upon a disease of the reasoning powers. Yet it is obvious that the mental processes in question are non-rational in the sense that they do not satisfy the laws of logic. The conclusions of the politician are not reached by impartially weighing the evidence before him; each step in his thinking is not the logical result of that which has preceded it. On the contrary, the conclusion is determined by the 'political-complex' present, and the evidence may be such that an unbiased application of logical principles would lead to a diametrically opposite result. We are forced to conclude, therefore, that in the domain where his 'political-complex' holds sway, the politician does not always think rationally, because his reasoning powers are not allowed free play. But he does not himself realise that his thoughts are logically vulnerable; they appear to him as propositions whose truth is at once obvious and beyond question, and he cannot understand how any other observer in possession of the same facts can possibly arrive at a different conclusion. 'To the Conservative, the amazing thing about the Liberal is his incapacity to see reason and accept the only possible solution of public problems.'[1]

The facts contained in the preceding paragraphs suggest further considerations which will enable us not only to correlate more exactly the mental processes of the insane with those occurring in normal men, but also to obtain an insight into the subjective aspect of the insane mind, that is to say, an insight into the abnormal mental processes as they appear to the patient himself.

There are, as a matter of fact, a large number of processes in the normal mind which possess those two characters, a non-rational origin and an immediate subjective obviousness, which are apparent in the case of the party politician or sectarian. The simplest instances are to be found in the thoughts and actions which are the direct result of the primary instincts, more particularly those of self-preservation, nutrition, and sex. William James says of them:

Science may come and consider these ways, and find that most of them are useful. But it is not for the sake of their utility that they are followed, but because at the moment of following them we feel that that is the only appropriate and natural thing to do. Not one man in a billion, when taking his dinner, ever thinks of utility. He eats because the food tastes good and makes him want more. If you ask him *why* he should want to eat more of what tastes like that, instead of revering you as a philosopher he will probably laugh at you for a fool. The connection between the savoury sensation and the act it awakens is for him absolute and *selbstverständlich*, an *a priori* synthesis of the most perfect sort, needing no proof but its own evidence. . . . To the metaphysician alone can such questions occur as: Why do we smile, when pleased, and not scowl? Why are we unable to talk to a crowd as we talk to a single

[1] W. Trotter, *Instincts of the Herd in Peace and War* (London, 1916).

friend? Why does a particular maiden turn our wits so upside down? The common man can only say, '*of course* we smile, *of course* our heart palpitates at the sight of a crowd, *of course* we love the maiden, that beautiful soul clad in that perfect form, so palpably and flagrantly made from all eternity to be loved!' And so probably does each animal feel about the particular things it tends to do in presence of particular objects. . . . To the broody hen the notion would probably seem monstrous that there should be a creature in the world to whom a nestful of eggs was not the utterly fascinating and precious and never-to-be-too-much-sat-upon object it is to her.

Trotter, in the extremely suggestive and stimulating articles upon 'Herd Instinct', from which we have quoted above, has shown that there is a vast group of mental processes possessing this same subjective aspect, although they do not arise from the three instincts commonly designated as primary. The assumptions, for example, 'upon which is based the bulk of opinion in matters of Church and State, the family, justice, probity, honour, purity, crime, and so forth' are characterised by this introspectual quality of the '*a priori* synthesis of the most perfect sort'. Trotter demonstrates that these are all the result of a fourth instinct, whose manifestations are of funda-mental importance in the psychology of gregarious animals, and to which he gives the name of 'herd instinct'.[1] Herd instinct ensures that the behaviour of the individual shall be in harmony with that of the community as a whole. Owing to its action each individual tends to accept without question the beliefs which are current in his class, and to carry out with unthinking obedience the rules of conduct upon which the herd has set its sanction. For the average man herd instinct is the force which determines his ethical code and all those beliefs and opinions which are not the result of a special knowledge. He carries out certain rules of life because his

[1] The psychoanalytical school does not accept Trotter's 'herd instinct' as a psychological entity, but regards it as a biological conception which does not correspond to any factor capable of being elicited by psychological analysis. According to this school, the phenomena which Trotter explains by herd instinct are the product of other instinctive forces, particularly those concerned in the relation of the developing individual to his parents.

fellow-men carry out these same rules; he believes certain things because he lives in an environment where those things are believed by everyone around him. If he is asked to explain his conduct or his opinions, he will, of course, at once produce rationalisations of the type we have described in chapter v and will persuade himself that these rationalisations are the actual causes of his behaviour. But in reality the causes responsible for his behaviour are, first, the fact that other people behave in that way, and secondly, the operation of herd instinct. The rationalisation is produced subsequently, and simply because man has an overwhelming need to believe that he is acting upon rational grounds.

If we examine the mental furniture of the average man, we shall find it made up of a vast number of judgments of a very precise kind upon subjects of very great variety, complexity, and difficulty. He will have fairly settled views upon the origin and nature of the universe, and upon what he will probably call its meaning; he will have conclusions as to what is to happen to him at death and after, as to what is and what should be the basis of conduct. He will know how the country should be governed, and why it is going to the dogs; why this piece of legislation is good, and that bad. He will have strong views upon military and naval strategy, the principles of taxation, the use of alcohol and vaccination, the treatment of influenza, the prevention of hydrophobia, upon municipal trading, the teaching of Greek, upon what is permissible in art, satisfactory in literature, and hopeful in science.

The bulk of such opinions must necessarily be without rational basis, since many of them are concerned with problems admitted by the expert to be still unsolved, while as to the rest it is clear that the training and experience of no average man can qualify him to have any opinion upon them at all. The rational method adequately used would have told him that on the great majority of these questions there could be for him but one attitude—that of suspended judgment.[1]

All these non-rational opinions and beliefs appear to their possessor as propositions whose truth is immediately obvious, and whose validity it is silly to question or to doubt. They are

[1] W. Trotter, *Instincts of the Herd in Peace and War* (London, 1916).

held, moreover, with a peculiar emotional warmth and instinctive certainty, which it is difficult to define, but whose character will be at once appreciated by anyone with a reasonable capacity for self-introspection. Genuine knowledge, the product of a scientific deduction from observed facts, appears in quite other guise than this. It is relatively cold, and devoid of the warmth which accompanies non-rational beliefs. If its truth is called in question we are not annoyed, but are merely stimulated to examine with renewed attention the foundations upon which it rests. The distinction between the two classes of mental process will be immediately apparent to the reader if he will compare, as regards their introspective aspect, his views upon the proposition that a man who ill-treats a woman is a cad, with his attitude to the proposition that the earth goes round the sun.

If these facts are considered in the light of the principles enunciated in foregoing chapters we shall easily recognise that non-rational beliefs and opinions are the product of complexes, and that the peculiar warmth we have described is the emotional tone which invariably accompanies the action of a complex. If we argue with the holder of such beliefs the complex will protect itself by one of two defensive reactions. Either the arguments will be rejected as senseless or wicked, or a flood of rationalisations will be produced which invest the belief with a plausibility entirely satisfactory to their creator.

Now these are precisely the characters which have been shown to exist in the delusions of the insane. They also have a non-rational origin, and are in reality the product of complexes. They also are accompanied by a peculiar emotional warmth, and a feeling of instinctive certainty. Moreover, they have to the patient himself just that same character of immediate obviousness and unquestionable truth, so that he cannot understand how we can fail to see how absolutely justifiable his contentions are, and how all the evidence makes the conclusions he has reached the only ones possible or conceivable.

This latter statement contains the answer to the problem posed upon a former page, the problem of representing to ourselves the subjective aspect of a delusion, the light in which the delusion must appear to the patient who possesses it. It appears as an obvious proposition, which none but the perverse can doubt, and which is so patently true that to attack it is only unprofitably silly or wicked.

We must therefore conclude that the insane patient is not irrational in the sense that his reasoning powers are in themselves different from those of normal men. It is true that certain of his mental processes have a non-rational origin, but it is equally true that the great bulk of opinions and beliefs held by the normal man arise in a similar way, and we cannot therefore on this account attribute a peculiar irrationality to the insane.

We are therefore faced with a further problem. If the position taken up in this chapter is correct, and if irrationality is not the hall-mark of insanity, what are the essential characters which distinguish the insane from the normal man? It must be confessed that in the present state of knowledge we can offer no completely satisfactory answer to this question, but our failure is due, in part at least, to the indefinite and almost meaningless nature of the problem presented to us. The terms employed therein have no precise significance, and of such terms it is obviously impossible to predicate any essential characters whatever. Insanity is not a definite entity like scarlet fever or tuberculosis, but it is used to denote a heterogeneous group of phenomena which have but little in common. Moreover, its boundaries have varied from age to age according to the dominating conceptions of the period, and it will be remembered that in chapter I we saw that individuals who in medieval times were regarded with esteem and reverence would now be removed without hesitation to a mental hospital.

All this being taken into account, the only solution of the problem which it seems feasible to offer consists in the mere enumeration of certain vague distinctions. No single one can be regarded as essential, but, taken in their entirety, they serve roughly to mark off the sphere of insanity from that of sanity.

The first criterion depends upon the degree in which the phenomena are manifested. We have endeavoured to demonstrate in preceding chapters that the symptoms of insanity are the result of psychological mechanisms which are identical with those found in the normal mind. In the former, however, the processes are carried to a more advanced stage, and beyond the limits which are generally regarded as normal. Thus the incompetent workman who ascribes his failure to the inferiority of his tools and the unfair treatment meted out to him by his employer is admittedly still sane, while the man who complains to the police that he is the victim of an organised boycott is certified to be suffering from 'delusions of persecution' and is removed to a hospital. In both cases the psychological mechanism is the same, but in the latter the process has been carried further.

Closely connected with this exaggeration which forms our first criterion is the second, and probably the most important, distinction between insanity and sanity, the distinction of conduct. The conduct of the insane is generally anti-social, and it is this criterion, expressed in the legal definition 'dangerous to himself or others', which in most cases determines whether or not the patient shall be sent to a mental hospital. The anti-social attribute which generally belongs to insane conduct may be positive or negative in character. Thus a patient may have persecutory delusions which make him an actual danger to his fellows, or which lead him to take his own life. On the other hand his behaviour may be anti-social in the sense that he is incapable of efficiently taking part in the social machine, as in the variety of insanity which we have termed 'emotional dementia'.

Other criteria depend upon the character of the psychological mechanisms responsible for the symptoms present. We have seen that many mental processes commonly met with in everyday life, as well as certain symptoms definitely regarded as insane, are due to the indirect manifestations of repressed complexes. In the latter group, however, the complex expression is generally more indirect, and therefore more distorted.

Associated with this is the further distinction that the rationalisations produced in the insane cases are as a rule more obvious and less plausible than those observed in everyday life.

The delusions of the insane resemble many of the beliefs and opinions held by the sane in the fact that in both cases the mental processes have a non-rational origin. In other respects, however, they differ to such an extent that it is generally easy to decide to which of the two groups a given symptom must be assigned. The beliefs of the sane, whether true or false, are generally supported by the opinion of a class, and are the result of the operation of herd instinct. The delusions of the insane, on the other hand, are not so supported, but are individual aberrations dependent upon factors working in direct opposition to herd instinct. This latter distinction is of great importance, and will be further considered in chapter XII. The beliefs of the sane, again, are often incompatible with facts, but no belief can be held for long which is very obviously contradicted by experience. For example, it is impossible for a sane pauper to believe that he is a millionaire. In the insane, however, we have seen that this gross incompatibility with experience is frequently observed. Moreover, although in normal men beliefs dependent upon strong emotional prejudices are apparently insusceptible to argument and to any but the most flagrant contradictions presented by actual experience, yet this insusceptibility is not absolute. The opposing forces exert a slow erosive effect which in process of time produces a gradual alteration in the belief, and perhaps ultimately destroys it. An insane delusion, however, seems altogether fixed and immune to this action, and the processes described only serve to elaborate the defences with which it is hedged round. All these latter distinctions depend upon the cardinal factor of dissociation. In the insane dissociation has been carried to a degree which is incompatible with normal thought or behaviour, and mental processes are allowed to pursue their course altogether undisturbed by the contradictions presented by the facts of experience.

CHAPTER XI

PHANTASY

THE normal effect of a complex is to produce action. A train of activity is set in motion whose goal is the realisation of the desires and tendencies constituting the driving force of the complex. The complex finds a complete expression in the achieving of its ends. There is, however, another mode of expression by which satisfaction is often obtained, although that satisfaction is only partial and limited. This second mode of expression is the construction of phantasy. In phantasy—or, to use the more widely known term, day-dreaming—we do not seek to satisfy our complexes in the world of reality, but content ourselves with the building of pleasant mental pictures in which the complexes attain an imaginary fulfilment.

The distinction between these two modes, the direct and complete expression in action, and the partial expression in phantasy, may be clearly seen in the effects produced by the so-called 'self-assertion complexes'. By the self-assertion complexes we mean those tendencies to aggrandisement of the self and the achieving of distinction amongst one's fellows which may be roughly grouped together under the heading of 'ambition'. Their normal direct effect is to be seen in the individual's struggle to get on, and to obtain a position which will ensure to him the respect and admiration of others. In addition to the direct expression in action, however, these complexes may expend a variable portion of their energy in the construction of phantasy. The phantasy produced in this way constitutes the common phenomenon of 'day-dreaming', which, although it occurs at every age, attains its most luxuriant development during adolescence. At this period the young man will often revel in astonishing feats of the imagination, fascinating scenes of great deeds and applauding crowds, in which, of course, he invariably plays the part of the hero.

In the construction of this imagery the complexes we have mentioned are assisted by the sex complexes, and the effects of the two causal groups are closely intermingled. The great deeds are generally performed before the admiring eyes of some fair lady whose favour the hero covets.

We do not hear much about these day-dreams, because their author is generally rather ashamed of his creations; in other words, they are subjected to a certain degree of that repression we have formerly described. Unless they are kept within reasonable bounds their influence must, indeed, be regarded as harmful, because the energy of the complexes is expended in the weaving of phantasies, and is not translated into action. This is the thought which underlies the following remarks of William James:

The weeping of a Russian lady over the fictitious personages in the play, while her coachman is freezing to death on his seat outside, is the sort of thing that everywhere happens on a less glaring scale. Even the habit of excessive indulgence in music, for those who are neither performers themselves nor musically gifted enough to take it in a purely intellectual way, has probably a relaxing effect upon the character. One becomes filled with emotions which habitually pass without prompting to any deed, and so the inertly sentimental condition is kept up. The remedy would be, never to suffer oneself to have an emotion at a concert without expressing it afterwards in some actual way. Let the expression be the least thing in the world—speaking genially to one's aunt, or giving up one's seat in a horse-car, if nothing more heroic offers—but let it not fail to take place.

The possibly pernicious effect of day-dreaming is seen even better when it is employed as a refuge, so to speak, from reality. If the young man we have described, in his efforts to make a career and to achieve distinction, experiences rebuffs and failures, he may be induced to allow his complexes to express themselves by the construction of phantasies rather than by the sterner struggle to alter facts. He may console himself by pleasant dreams in which he marches to imaginary victories, while his enemies bow the knee in envious admiration. He may live for a time in so attractive a world that he finds it hard to drag himself back into relation with things as they are. In our technical language we should say that he finds the complex incompatible with his actual environment, that there is a conflict between the complex and reality. He compromises with the difficulty by making no further attempts to combine the two opposing forces, but gives up the struggle with life, and retires temporarily into a world of the imagination where the complex works its will without colliding against brutal facts.

This phenomenon is extremely common, and most of us at one time or another console ourselves for the failure of our ambitions in the real world by the creation of these pleasant fancies. But a path opens here which leads us easily across the bridge into the regions of insanity, and the processes just considered provide a key to the interpretation of many of the symptoms which we observe in the mental hospital.

In the normal cases the individual is aware that he is day-dreaming, and does not altogether lose touch with the real world. His friends observe that he is 'absent-minded' and absorbed in his own ideas, and that he takes no notice of what goes on around him. But he is able if necessary to drag himself back into relation with the actual environment, although to do so often requires an appreciable effort. In other words, he is dissociated to some extent from the realities of everyday life, but this dissociation is only partial, incomplete, and temporary. If, however, the process assumes proportions which are definitely morbid, this dissociation becomes more pronounced and permanent. The patient, as he may now be called, separates himself altogether from the real world and devotes all his mental energy to day-dreaming. He lives permanently in a self-made world where all the desires and ambitions belonging to the complex are luxuriantly fulfilled. This mechanism is responsible for the symptoms observed in two types of insanity which, although closely allied to one another, may be roughly separated for descriptive purposes.

The first type, which may be regarded as an exaggeration of normal day-dreaming, comprises a number of those cases grouped in chapter III under the heading of 'emotional dementia'. The patient has apparently lost all interest in life; he expresses no desires or ambitions, makes no effort to employ himself in any way, and sits from day to day in the same corner of the ward, inert and lethargic. His face is vacant and expressionless, and he seems oblivious of everything which takes place around him. If he is addressed he will perhaps vouchsafe a monosyllabic reply, but it is impossible to rouse him from his apathy, and he will receive the news of his parents' deaths with the same untroubled equanimity with which he eats his dinner. To the casual observer such a patient appears to have lost all mental activity, but, if we examine his mind more closely and look below its congealed surface, we find that activity still exists, although it is diverted into channels which lead to no external manifestation or practical result. All the available energy is absorbed in the construction of pleasant phantasies of the kind we have described. The patient has retired altogether into a world of day-dreams, and for him the facts of real life have lost all significance and interest.

In the second type the patient has immersed himself in his imaginary world even more completely and efficiently. The phantasy created by his own mind acquires the tang of actual reality: he believes that he *is* the conquering hero or the multi-millionaire, and that the pleasant pictures he once imagined have become the facts of life. He has crossed the barrier which separates in the normal man day-dreams from the dreams that accompany sleep, and the creations of an idle fancy have become the delusions of insanity. A further degree of dissociation has been attained, and the complexes achieve a luxuriant expression undisturbed by the flagrant contradictions which experience everywhere presents to them.

This mechanism, which has been termed 'wish fulfilment', furnishes a psychological interpretation for a vast number of the manifestations of insanity. One of the simplest examples of its action is seen in the so-called 'betrothal-delirium', occasionally to be observed in women who have been jilted. All the desires and ambitions which hitherto formed the kernel of the patient's life have suddenly become incompatible with reality.

Out of the intense emotional stress engendered by this conflict a condition of insanity develops, characterised by a dream-like delirium in which the frustrated complexes attain an imaginary fulfilment. In this delirium the patient believes that she has been reconciled to her lover, preparations for the wedding are in progress, the bridegroom arrives, the marriage ceremony takes place, and the dream-state is prolonged indefinitely in pictures of a subsequent wedded life, each of which is lived through with all the intensity of reality.

In other cases the symptoms are less dramatic in character, but essentially similar in their mode of origin. A system of morbid mental processes develops in which the complexes that have been denied expression in the world of reality obtain a delusional fulfilment. The patient believes that the defaulting lover has returned to his allegiance, or perhaps that she has actually become his wife. The obvious inconsistency of such beliefs with the real facts of life is glossed over by the production of suitable rationalisations, and the development of those secondary delusions which have already been described on p. 71.

A similar mechanism accounts for those complicated and fantastic delusional systems which characterise a large percentage of the cases met with in the chronic wards of the hospital. Thus one of my patients announces that she is descended from Queen Elizabeth, and is herself the rightful queen of England. She has been given the title of 'Rule Britannia', has several armies under her control, and is at the moment engaged in issuing orders to her generals to make a combined attack upon all the nations of Europe. She complains bitterly, however, that her movements are hampered by a conspiracy directed by 'Mr Guelph', who has succeeded in obtaining her incarceration in an asylum, and who strives to rob her of all the privileges which belong to her rank.

This patient, prior to the outbreak of her insanity, was a hard-working woman of the servant class, whose life had contained little but a constant succession of hardships. In the grandiose delusions which she exhibits, the day-dreams of the class that thrives on cheap romantic literature may easily be recognised, now elevated by a process of dissociation to the rank of an actual belief, and pursuing their course in a logic-tight compartment secure from the contradiction of facts. Protected in this way from the controlling influence of real experience, the self-assertion complexes strive to achieve a luxuriant expression by the production of constantly elaborated phantasies of grandeur. The persecutory ideas concerning the conspiracy, on the other hand, are to be regarded as the secondary delusions which generally arise in such cases as processes of rationalisation.

In all these cases the final outbreak of insanity occurs as the solution of a conflict. The patient is unable to achieve his ambitions, either because the environment opposes insurmountable obstacles or because his capacities are not equal to his desires—in other words, there is a conflict between the complex and reality. This conflict is avoided by allowing the complex to obtain a partial expression by the construction of phantasy, while the incompatibility of the real world is masked by the production of the requisite degree of dissociation. Under such circumstances it might be said that reality is repressed, while the complex plays unchecked upon the surface of consciousness.

There is, however, another method by which conflict may be avoided in these cases, equally morbid in its character and effects. If the patient finds that the complex cannot be satisfied in the world of reality he may endeavour to banish it altogether from his life, to forget that he has ever experienced those particular desires, and to behave as if they had never existed. In other words he remains in touch with reality, and strives to repress the complex.

These two methods of dealing with an intolerable conflict frequently occur in the same patient, and both are well illustrated in the following case, originally described by Jung.[1]

A man of between thirty and forty years of age, of exceptional intelligence, and an archaeologist of note, was brought

[1] C. G. Jung, *Der Inhalt der Psychose* (Vienna, 1908).

to the hospital in a condition of acute maniacal excitement. He was of short stature, thin and weakly, and he stuttered abominably. His history was as follows: He had been an intellectually precocious boy, and had early devoted himself to the study of archaeology, finishing his education at the University of B——. At the conclusion of his university career he buried himself altogether in the pursuit of science, cut himself off more and more from the world and from his friends, and finally led the life of a complete hermit. Some years later, while on a holiday tour, he returned to B——, where he spent most of his days in long walks among the outskirts of the town. After one of these excursions he complained of feeling nervous and restless. A state of excitement developed, passing rapidly into the acute delirium which led to his removal to the hospital. On admission he was intensely confused, had no idea where he was, and spoke only in short sentences which nobody understood. Periods of violent excitement were often present, during which he attacked all those about him, and could only be restrained by the united efforts of several attendants. Gradually the delirium abated, and one day the patient suddenly awoke as if from a long dream, rapidly returned to his normal condition, and was shortly afterwards discharged from the institution. He immediately resumed his former life, and in the following year produced several works of the first rank. His acquaintances only observed that he seemed more of a misanthrope and more of a hermit than ever. Then once again he came to B——, and again occupied his days in long walks. A fainting attack in the street was followed by an outbreak of delirium, and for the second time he was brought to the hospital. On this occasion, however, the symptoms were different from those noted during his former illness. He performed complicated gymnastics all over the room, spoke of his marvellous muscular power and bodily beauty, announced himself to be a great singer, and continually sang love ditties of his own composition. After a time the delirium lessened, he became more accessible, and it was possible for Dr Jung to undertake an analysis of the case.

If we now study the patient's history in the light of the facts revealed by that analysis, our understanding of the case will be considerably increased. During the time when the patient was a student in B—— he fell in love with a certain lady, and they were in the habit of taking long walks in the neighbourhood of the town. The shyness and feeling of shame of the stutterer prevented him from declaring his passion, and, moreover, marriage was at that time a financial impossibility. At the end of his university career he left B——, and never again saw the lady. Shortly afterwards he heard that she had married somebody else. Then he buried himself in his hermit's life, and strove to forget; in other words, the complex, painful through its incompatibility with reality, was repressed. We have seen, however, that, though a complex may be repressed, it does not thereby cease to exist. It disappears from consciousness, and is not allowed to play its normal part in the thoughts and activity of the mind. But it persists underneath, as it were, and sooner or later it manifests itself by one of those indirect methods which we have dealt with in former chapters. This is what actually occurred in the case we are describing.

We saw that after some years of strenuous work our patient returned to the town of B——, and that a few days later the first outbreak of delirium occurred. The explanation of this delirium is simple—the repressed complex had burst on to the surface. The content of the patient's mind during the attack may be described as follows: He found himself in the chaos of a mighty dream; great battles were in progress, and he was always in the centre of the fight, performing prodigies of valour and leading the armies with marvellous skill, while the lady watched and awaited him as the prize of victory. This was the period when he blindly attacked all those about him and struggled furiously with his attendants. Then came the final victory—the bride approached, and he awoke once more to reality and the dull routine of his life. The complex was again repressed.

It will be observed how closely the content of this delirium resembles the ordinary adolescent day-dreaming which we have previously described. The difference consists merely in a degree of dissociation which permits the complex to manifest itself in a definitely hallucinatory form, altogether cut loose from the control of the personality.

In the second attack, which, like the first, was preceded by a visit to B——, the course of events was somewhat different. The complexes which then manifested themselves, although obviously closely allied to the sex complex, were rather those which had arisen as a result of his bodily infirmities. It will be remembered that he was stunted and unattractive, his muscles atrophied and weak, and that he stuttered abominably. He was entirely unmusical, his voice was harsh, and he was incapable of singing a note in tune. All this formed part of a complex of bodily shame, which we saw in action at the time he was courting his lady. Coupled with it, of course, was the intense secret desire that the defects could be removed. During the second attack of delirium this was the complex which emerged to the surface, with all its desires fictitiously fulfilled. He was immensely strong, and a gymnast of the first rank—hence the complicated antics he performed around the room. He was the greatest singer in the world, and a prodigious orator. He possessed, in fact, the corresponding virtue for every defect which reality had inflicted upon him.

The psychological interpretation of this case may therefore be resumed as follows. The complex is incompatible with reality, and the patient gives up the attempt to reconcile the two. At intervals he abandons reality and plunges into the complex—or, as it has been expressed, he flies into the disease to obtain a refuge from reality. During the periods which intervene between the outbreaks of delirium he adopts another method of solving the conflict. He preserves his grasp on the external world and avoids the conflict by the process of repressing the complex. But this can only be done at the cost of annihilating a whole segment of his emotional life, and he becomes a misanthrope and a hermit.

In many chronic cases, as in the example described upon p. 110, these so-called periods of sanity, during which the incompatible complex is successfully repressed, are absent. The patient retires altogether into the complex and lives permanently in a self-made world where all the desires and ambitions belonging to the complex are luxuriantly fulfilled. Under such circumstances the complex frequently undergoes a process known as 'degradation'. The phraseology in which it finds expression becomes more distorted and stereotyped, often degenerating into a meaningless hotch-potch of words, and the mental processes generated by the complex become concentrically diminished. Finally, the whole mental life of the patient consists, perhaps, in the performance of some single stereotyped action representing the wreck of the old complex. The patient described on p. 88, who spent her whole existence in the sewing of an imaginary boot, furnishes an excellent example of this terminal stage.

The degradation of speech and mental content proceeds according to fairly precise laws which have been laboriously investigated by Jung and his followers. Space does not permit of any further description of them here, but it may be said that by their aid it is possible to show that even the most incoherent and apparently meaningless speech has nevertheless a definite significance, capable of being elucidated by psychological analysis.

There is one further psychological process which may profitably be dealt with in the present chapter, as it is intimately related to the phantasy construction to which our attention has so far been devoted. This process, technically known as 'identification', is of considerable importance, and in its minor degrees is frequently manifested in normal mental life. It consists in identifying ourselves with another individual, either real or fictitious, so that we experience his joys, sorrows, and desires, as if they were our own. So long as the identification holds we feel that he is part of our personality, and that we are living part of our lives in him. Identification is frequently encountered in both normal and abnormal psychology—it includes many of the phenomena generally grouped under the heading of 'sympathy'. The meaning of the conception will be made clearer by the consideration of some illustrative examples. One of the best instances is afforded by the reader of a second-rate romantic novel. The explanation of the interest which this type of fiction arouses lies in the fact that the reader identifies himself with the hero, lives with him through a series of astonishing adventures, falls in love with the heroine, and lives happily ever afterwards. The novel, in fact, permits the reader to experience the fascinations of day-dreaming without the trouble of constructing the imagery himself.

An even better example is presented by the audience of a melodrama. Everybody who has observed the gallery during an entertainment of this kind is aware that its inmates are living on the stage, and always, of course, in the part of the hero or heroine. The illusion of reality which attaches to the play allows the day-dreaming to be conducted much more efficiently than in the case of the novel—hence the greater popularity of the drama. It is because the audience insists that its day-dreaming should be catered for, that the playwright is compelled to provide a liberal supply of peers, and to cast his scenes not too far from Mayfair.

If we rise higher in the scale of art and consider the first-rate novel or play, we find the mechanism of identification still at work, but appearing now in a less simple form. The reader no longer identifies himself merely with the hero, but rather with all the characters at once. He finds portrayed the complexes, or partial tendencies, which exist in his own mind—and in the action of the novel he reads the conflicts and struggles which he experiences in his own life. Precisely the same remarks are applicable to the first-rate play. The reason that such productions only appeal to a limited class is that they presuppose in their audience the possession of mental processes sufficiently complicated to enable this identification to occur. It must be clearly understood, of course, that we are making no attempt to reduce all the psychological phenomena produced by the novel and play to this single mechanism, but only to trace out one of the factors on which these works of art depend.

The mechanism of identification underlies many anomalous

actions of whose real origin the individual himself is altogether unconscious. One of my patients became involved without apparent reason in a lawsuit which an acquaintance was bringing against his wife. He plunged into the case with extraordinary zeal, entirely neglected his own business, supplied his acquaintance with considerable funds, and did everything that was possible to further the latter's victory. When I inquired the reason of his behaviour, he assured me that he was actuated solely by friendship and by a love of abstract justice. In this, of course, the process which we have formerly described as rationalisation will be easily recognised. Investigation showed that the alleged friendship was only of a few weeks' standing, and that abstract justice was very obviously on the opposite side. The real cause of my patient's action was found by psychological analysis to be that he was himself engaged in a bitter dispute with his own wife. He had therefore unconsciously identified himself with the other man, who happened to be in a similar situation. The same mechanism may be observed in the example described on p. 61, of the patient who was so disturbed at the ill-treatment inflicted upon two foreigners.

The stimulus which gives rise to the identification is often to be found in the fact that the second individual possesses some character or environment which is coveted by the first. This is seen in a simple form in the play of the child who 'pretends' to be 'father', and thereby achieves the magical joys of being grown up. A more complicated variety of the same process plays a prominent part in the causation of many hysterical symptoms. The numerous ills which occur in these cases are frequently the result of unconscious identification with a second individual who is afflicted with an organic disease, but who also has some other character which is strenuously desired by the patient. An hysterical patient of my own, for example, suffered from severe attacks of vertigo—analysis showed that his symptoms were entirely the result of identification with his father, who was the subject of chronic ear-disease, an affection often associated with vertigo.

Identification is intimately bound up with those day-dreaming processes which have been dealt with in the earlier portion of the present chapter. The day-dreamer who witnesses the triumphal progress of some popular hero through the streets lives himself into the part of the central figure, and marches with him through the cheering crowds. From this simple and well-known phenomenon a chain of allied manifestations leads finally to the chronic wards of the hospital, where we encounter a most distinguished assemblage of emperors, generals, and other representatives of the great.

CHAPTER XII

THE SIGNIFICANCE OF CONFLICT

IF we now review the field which we have surveyed in the present volume, and consider the implements which have proved of value in the investigation of its details, we shall at once observe that there are two of those implements which have been pressed into service at almost every turn. These are the conceptions of dissociation and conflict, and their utility has been so great that it will be profitable to examine from a more comprehensive and general point of view the part which they play in mental life.

We have seen that a vast number of abnormal phenomena, ranging from hallucinations and delusions to the complicated phantasy productions described in the last chapter, are to be regarded as examples of dissociation. The mind has lost that homogeneity which is the ideal of the normal personality, and has become disintegrated into more or less independent portions, each pursuing its own course and development without reference to the welfare of the whole.

We have seen, moreover, that this disintegration has invariably owed its existence to the presence of a conflict. Homogeneity has disappeared because the mind contains elements which are incompatible with each other, and dissociation has arisen as a method of avoiding the storm and stress which the warring of these mutually hostile elements would otherwise inevitably produce. Dissociation is therefore to be regarded biologically as a refuge from the stress of conflict, and as one of nature's methods of dealing with conflicts which seem insoluble by other means. Hence, if we would investigate the causes responsible for abnormal mental phenomena, the discovery that dissociation exists is only the first step in the process, and it is always necessary to pass further back to the conflict which will be found behind it.

Conflict, therefore, would seem to be a fundamental factor in the causation of mental disorder, and the determination of its precise significance a problem of prime importance for psychology and for science. At present the full significance of conflict is imperfectly understood, and any general discussion of the subject must therefore be largely speculative in character. It will, nevertheless, bé of interest to consider shortly the deductions that may be drawn with some degree of confidence from the knowledge so far gained, and the directions in which it would seem profitable to prosecute further research.

In the former chapters of this book our task has generally been the elucidation of some individual symptom, and we have therefore not attempted to push the analysis of the patient's mental condition further than was necessary for this purpose. Hence in most cases the conflict which we have discovered to be immediately responsible for the genesis of the symptom has been of a comparatively minor character, and the complexes concerned have involved only the more superficial elements of the mind.

When, however, a more profound analysis has been made, and the investigation has been carried sufficiently far to explain the origin of the whole mental state, a conflict of a more fundamental character has finally been unearthed. This fundamental conflict involves factors of an importance commensurate with the effects produced, and generally leads us back to the great primary instincts which constitute the principal driving forces of the mind. We find a struggle taking place in which one of these primary instincts is pitted against another, or in which the desires and tendencies arising from such an instinct are opposed and thwarted by conditions enforced upon the patient by his environment and circumstances. It may therefore be concluded that in conflicts of these two types are probably to be found the essential causes responsible for many of the manifestations of mental disorder.

Freud considered that the origin of all cases belonging to certain varieties of mental disease can be traced back to factors connected with a single one of the great instincts, that of sex. We should expect, of course, that the immense power of the sex impulses, and the opposition which inevitably arises between them and the rules of conduct imposed by civilised society, would make this instinct one of the most prevalent sources of conflict and mental disintegration. Nevertheless, Freud's generalisation has not been universally accepted and, even allowing for the fact that Freud's conception of sex is far wider than is covered by the ordinary use of the term, it is perhaps safer at the present time to assume that the conflicts in question may involve factors connected with any of the fundamental instinctive forces of the mind, provided that these factors are of sufficient emotional intensity. We shall readily admit that sex probably plays a predominant part in a majority of cases, but shall be prepared to find that a certain number are dependent upon conflicts in which other mental elements are mainly concerned.

Among the great primary instincts which provide the opposing forces responsible for mental conflict a dominant place must be assigned to 'herd instinct'.[1] It has been explained in chapter x (p. 100) that a vast part of the beliefs and conduct of man is due to the operation of this instinct. From it the tendencies generally ascribed to tradition and to education derive most of their power. It provides the mechanism by which the ethical code belonging to a particular class is enforced upon each individual member of that class, so that the latter is instinctively impelled to think and to act in the manner which the code prescribes. That is to say, a line of conduct upon which the herd has set its sanction acquires all the characters of an instinctive action, although this line of conduct may have no rational basis, may run counter to the dictates of experience, and may be in direct opposition to the tendencies generated by the other primary instincts. This opposition to other primary instincts is well exemplified in the case of sex, where the impulses due to the latter are constantly baulked and controlled by the opposing tendencies arising from our moral education and tradition.

[1] Cf. footnote on p. 100.

It will be immediately obvious that in these struggles between the primary instincts and the beliefs and codes enforced by the operation of herd instinct we have a fertile field for the development of mental conflict. Each of the factors involved possesses an enormous emotional force, and we should therefore expect that their opposition would produce a plentiful crop of the abnormal mental phenomena described in the preceding chapters of this book. Trotter, who has fully developed the subject in the papers to which we have already frequently referred, has pointed out the immense significance which the conflict between primitive instinct and herd tradition possesses for the human mind. He remarks that the manifestations of mental disintegration thereby produced

are coming to be recognised over a larger and larger field, and in a great variety of phenomena. . . . This field includes a part of insanity, how much we cannot even guess, but certainly a very large part; it includes the group of conditions described as functional diseases of the nervous system, and, finally, it includes that vast group of the mentally unstable which, while difficult to define without detailed consideration, is sufficiently precise in the knowledge of all to be recognisable as extremely large.

In the last chapter we have described several cases in which the outbreak of insanity depended upon the existence of a conflict between the dominating complexes of the mind and the circumstances in which the individual was compelled to live. It was shown that the abnormal phenomena finally produced could be regarded as biological reactions whose purpose was to provide a way of escape from the strain of this intolerable struggle. The individual found a refuge in dissociation, and retired into an imaginary world where the complexes attained a delusional fulfilment, while all the mental processes incompatible with this imaginary world were shut out of the field of consciousness. Now in cases of this type it is interesting to note that among the processes thus excluded from effectual participation in consciousness are to be found almost all the tendencies due to the operation of herd instinct.

The patients have lost the gregarious attributes of the normal man, and the sanctions of traditional conduct have no longer any significance for them. In the milder cases this change shows itself merely as a loss of interest in the affairs of their fellows, a tendency to be solitary and unsociable, an atrophy of their affections for friends and relatives, and an indifference to the ordinary conventions of society. In the advanced cases the change is much more marked, and the mind is completely withdrawn from participation in the life of the herd. The code of conduct imposed by convention and traditions no longer regulates the patient's behaviour, and he becomes slovenly, filthy, degraded, and shameless. In this picture, to which so many chronic patients conform, may be recognised the absolute negation of herd instinct and of the vast group of mental activities which arise therefrom.

These facts suggest the hypothesis that the fundamental mechanism which underlies this vast group of the insanities consists essentially in a dissociation of herd instinct. It is possible that the individual who is faced with an intolerable conflict between his primitive instincts on the one hand, and his environment and traditions on the other, and who has found a refuge by retiring into a world of phantasy and shutting out the world of reality, can only achieve this by dissociating herd instinct from the other primary forces of the mind and refusing to allow it any longer to play a part therein. If this hypothesis should prove to be correct, prevention would resolve itself into the problem of how to obviate the underlying dissociation. In order to achieve this it would be necessary to deal with the conflict which had produced it, and the remedy would lie in attacking one or other of the antagonists so that incompatibility no longer existed. The primitive instincts cannot presumably be altered, and the attack would therefore have to be directed either against the traditions and codes which obtain their force from the operation of herd instinct or, naturally more hopefully, against the particular ways in which those traditions and codes are acting upon the mind of the patient. It may be possible to modify these so that the flagrant incompatibilities which produce these disastrous consequences are no longer produced.

How far measures of this kind can be applied to those gross disturbances which we have latterly been considering is highly speculative, but there can be no doubt that minor mental disorders, which are dependent upon conflicts of an essentially similar character, though much less in degree, can be profitably attacked along this road. Modern psychotherapy, which has advanced greatly since this book was first written, has shown how much can be achieved in this way.

INDEX

Action, stereotyped, 37, 38
Activities, simultaneous, 41
Adler, A., viii, 12
Ajax, 15
Alcoholism, 84, 92
Alterations in speech, 37
Amnesia, 33
Anaesthesia, hysterical, 4, 17
Apathy, 30, 32
Argument, imperviousness to, 97, 98
Association experiment, 59, 60
Astronomy, development of, 22
Atomic theory, 23
Auditory hallucinations, 34
Automatic writing, 42, 43

Beliefs, non-rational, 98 ff.
Betrothal-delirium, 109
Bias, party, 56
Bourne, Rev. Ansel, 46
Brahe, Tycho, 22
Breur, Josef, 3

Censure, 78, 81 ff.
Cerebral topography, 19
Charcot, 1
Complex; Complexes, 26, 54 ff.
  bias, 55
  normal action of, 54 ff.
  political, 56, 57, 60, 98
  repressed, action of, 78 ff.
Conceptions of mental disorder, 15
  demonological, 16, 18
  physiological, 4, 18, 19, 24, 26
  political, 18
  psychological, 15, 20, 21 ff., 28
Concepts, 24
Conflict, 65 ff., 119 ff.
Conolly, 19
Conscious processes, 4, 25

Consciousness, 2
  dissociation of, 39 ff.
  field of, 40
Copernicus, 22
Cynicism, 84

Dalton, 23
Day-dreaming, 106 ff.
Deficiency, mental, 29, 39
Delusions, 34 ff., 97, 105
  fixity of, 35
  of grandeur, 34, 71, 110
  of persecution, 34, 35, 92
  of reference, 35, 94
  secondary, 71
Dementia, 30, 39
  emotional, 32, 40, 104, 108
  senile, 30
Depression, 30, 31, 40
Determinism, psychological, 53
Development of psychopathology, 1 ff.
Devil's claw, 17
Devine, 82
Dissociation, 2, 10, 39 ff., 105, 119
  of consciousness, 41 ff.
  the result of conflict, 68, 69
Double personality, 45, 46, 69, 76
Dreams, 5, 6, 7
Drunkard's humour, 83

Ego, 7, 47
  and libido, 7, 12
Emotional dementia, 32, 40, 104, 108
Esquirol, 19
Excitement, 30, 40
  manic, 31

Field of consciousness, 40
Fixation of libido, 7
Foreconscious, 5, 6

Forgetting, 73
Freud, vi, viii. 3 ff., 20, 36, 53, 120
  development of, 3 ff.
  sex theory of, 6, 7
Functional nervous disorders, 1

Grandiose delusions, 34, 71, 110

Hallucinations, 34, 69
  auditory, 34, 49
  tactile, 34
  visual, 34
Hanwell, 19
Heinroth, 20
Herd instinct, 100 ff., 121 ff.
Hippocrates, 16, 18
Hobbies, 54
Homer, mental disorders in, 15
Humanitarianism, development of,
  18, 19
Humour, 83
Hypnotism, 8
Hysteria, 1, 4, 5, 8, 42
Hysterical anaesthesia, 4, 17

Identification, 115 ff.
Insane, anti-social attribute of the,
  104
  irrationality of the, 96 ff.
Insanity
  demonological conception of, 16,
    18
  Hippocratic conception of, 16, 18
  old maids', 93
  physiological conception of, 18, 20
  projection in, 92
  psychological conception of, 15,
    20, 21 ff.
Instinct, herd, 100 ff., 121 ff.
Instincts, primary, 99, 100
Irène, case of, 33, 44, 45, 47, 74, 75,
  79
Irrationality of the insane, 96 ff.
Irritability, 62

James, William, 46, 99, 157
Janet, P., vi, 2, 20, 33

Jekyll and Hyde, 46
Jung, C. G., vi, viii, 8, 12, 20, 53,
  54, 59, 60, 61, 79, 88, 111, 115

Kepler, 22, 23
Kraepelin, 20
Krafft-Ebing, vi

Libido, 6, 7
  development of, 7 ff.
  phases of, 7
Logic-tight compartment, 50, 67,
  68, 69, 72, 73, 74

Magnetism, 1
Mania, washing, 36, 49, 84
Manic excitement, 31
McDougal, 54
Mechanisms, 5, 11
Medium, 15
Mental capacity, defects of, 29
  qualitative changes in, 30, 39
Mental deficiency, 29, 39
Mental disorders, history of, 15 ff.
  phenomena of, 28 ff.
Mental processes, unconscious, 26
Mesmer, 1
Mind, regions of, 5
Motor-area, 20
Mutism, 86

Nebuchadnezzar, 15
Nervous disorders, functional, 1
Neurasthenia, 1
Neurotic cases, 33
Non-rational beliefs, 101, 102

Obsession, 36, 48, 69
Old maid's insanity, 93
Old Testament, mental disorders in,
  15

Party bias, 56, 98
Pearson, Karl, vi, 22
Persecution, delusions of, 34 ff., 71,
  92, 93, 104

Personality, 47, 65
  double, 45, 46, 69, 76
Perversion, sexual, 7
Phantasy, 106 ff.
Phraseology, alterations in, 37
Pinel, 19
Prejudice, 91
Projection, 89, 90 ff.
Prudery, 81, 82, 93
Psychiatry, 19
Psychoanalysis, 8
  orthodox school of, 11, 37, 100
Psychological determinism, 53
Psychopathology, development of,
  1 ff., 10 ff.

Rationalisation, 57, 58, 70, 97
Reaction time, 59
Reaction word, 59
Reference, delusions of, 35, 94
Repressed complexes, action of,
  78 ff.
Repression, 4, 6, 26, 72 ff.
Resistance, 4

Sanity v. insanity, 103, 104, 105
Saul, 15
Science, method of, 21 ff.
Self-deception, 57

Self-reproach, 91, 94
Sentiment, 54
Sex, evolution of, 6, 7
Shand, 54
Shyness, 82
Somnambulism, 33, 44, 45, 46, 47,
  69, 74 ff., 79
Speech, alterations in, 37
Spes phthisica, 83
Spiritualism, 43
Stereotyped action, 37, 88
Suggestion, 1, 2
Symbolisation, 88
Sympathy, 115

Test, association, 59, 60
Topography, cerebral, 19
Trotter, W., vi, 85, 99, 100, 101, 122

Ulysses, 15
Unconscious mental processes, 4, 26
Unconscious region of mind, 4, 5, 6

Vorbeireden, 85

Washing mania, 36, 49, 84
Wish-fulfilment, 109
Witchcraft, 17
Writing, automatic, 42, 43

Bradford College Library

BF173 .H39 1957   BCHA
Hart, Bernard/The psychology of insanity

3 6660 00030 4641